The Natural Guide
to Great Sex

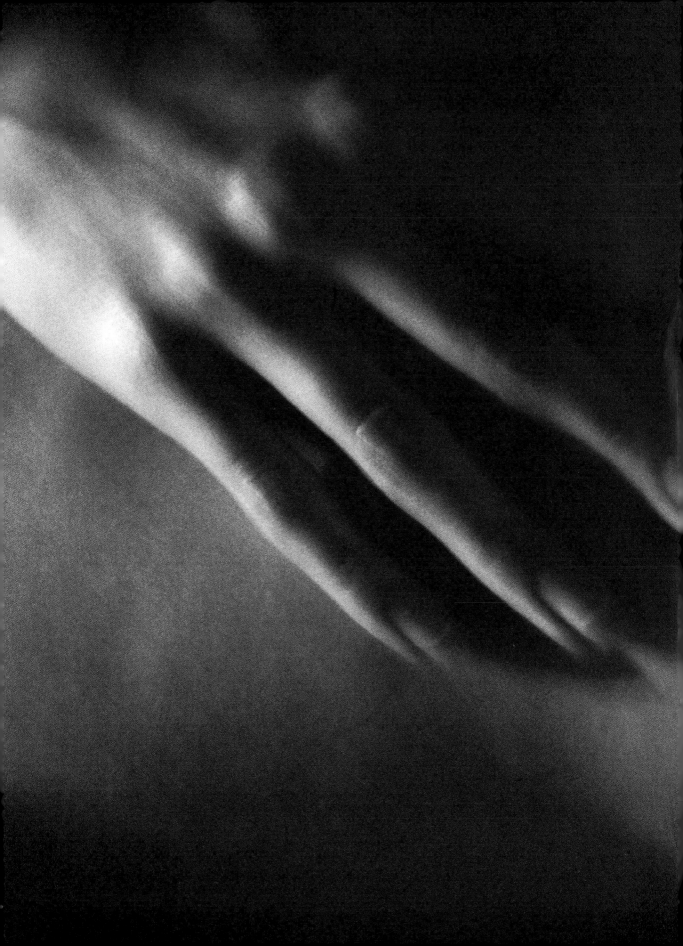

The Natural Guide
to Great Sex

Ellen Kamhi R.N., Ph.D.

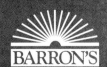

BARRON'S

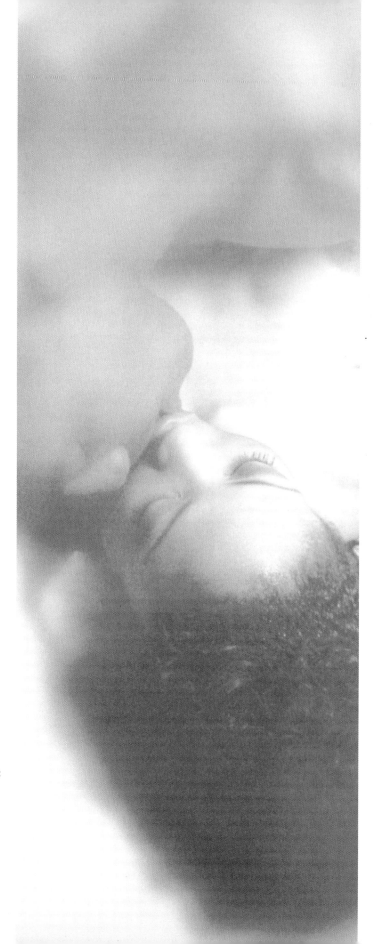

First edition for the United States and Canada published
in 2004 by Barron's Educational Series, Inc.

First published in Great Britain in 2004
by GODSFIELD PRESS LTD,
Laurel House, Station Approach,
Alresford, Hampshire SO24 9JH, U.K.
www.godsfieldpress.com

Project Designer: Lisa McCormick
Designer: John Grain
Project Editor: Susie Behar
Photographer: Alistair Hughes
Picture Researcher: Vanessa Fletcher

Designed and produced for Godsfield Press
by THE BRIDGEWATER BOOK COMPANY

All inquiries should be addressed to:
Barron's Educational Series, Inc.
250 Wireless Boulevard
Hauppauge, New York 11788
http://www.barronseduc.com

International Standard Book Number 0-7641-2631-8
Library of Congress Catalog Card Number 2003101020

Printed and bound in China
9 8 7 6 5 4 3 2 1

ATTENTION: The information included in this book
is for information purposes only. It is not intended to
be used as a basis for self-treatment or as a substitute for
professional medical care. The reader should consult a
qualified health professional in regard to all symptoms,
treatments, and dosage recommendations. Any reader
taking prescription medication must be especially careful
to seek professional medical attention before using any part
of the remedies described in this book. The author and
publisher disclaim any responsibility for adverse effects
related to the usage of any information presented in this
book. Any application of the information contained in this
book is at the reader's own discretion and risk.

Contents

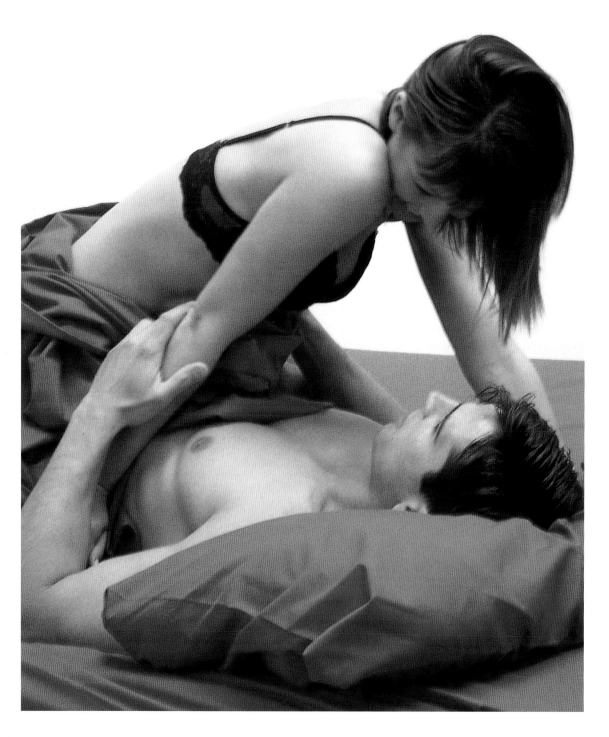

Introduction

The strong, overriding influence of sexuality has acted as a formative force in the lives of individuals and has influenced the course of entire civilizations. Humans are one of the few species known to use sex not only for procreation but also for recreation.[1] Views of sex range from a base indulgence in total hedonism to a loving embrace to the highest levels of spirituality and mysticism. The schizophrenic nature of humankind's struggle with the powerful sexual force can be seen in the attempts to both deify and totally repress sexuality. The voluptuous erotic sculptures and works of art that adorn the ancient Hindu temples of India reflect the divine bliss experienced at the instant of orgasm—sexual transcendence. In contrast, other religious teachings take great pains to cover all parts of the body with nonerotic apparel in an attempt to sublimate sexual nature.

Ancient beliefs, as well as modern science, support the notion that great sex directly relates to great overall health. Civilizations of old revered elder leaders, especially if they continued to produce offspring into their later years. Many older men and women enjoy sex into advanced age, and those who do report a high level of overall life satisfaction.

The Natural Guide to Great Sex delves into these ideas and takes a practical approach to a wide variety of natural methods that people can employ to further their knowledge of their own sexuality, to increase their sexual energy, and ultimately to enjoy a fulfilling sex life.

Chapter 1 begins with an explanation of hormones, those magical complex chemicals that need to be maintained in balance in order for sex to be successful. You'll learn the function of various hormones and how you can naturally maintain them at optimum levels.

In Chapter 2 you will explore foods, herbs, and supplements that have been used as aphrodisiacs throughout the ages.

Your love life is much more intricate than the interaction of hormones and nutrients. The energy between two people is paramount to initiating a sexual attraction. Chapter 3 delves into various techniques that can balance and "rev up" your interpersonal energy field, such as exercise, dance, and yoga, ancient Taoist exercises, and homeopathic and essence remedies.

Chapter 4 explores many ancient life-force energy-enhancing techniques for sexual bliss. Reclaim the mystical understanding of yin and yang from the Orient, ancient Indian teachings about tantra, Jewish mystical secrets of kabbalah, and the orgone energy teachings of Wilhelm Reich, a student of Sigmund Freud. Follow the easy instructions to make your own orgone accumulator.

In Chapter 5 you will experience titillating the sexual senses. Find out what your favorite color means in terms of your sexual self, and understand how rhythm can stimulate or sedate, according to the mysticism of vocalizations. Learn to share the touch of a sensual massage and breathe deeply as you explore the deliciously tantalizing world of aromatherapy.

Easy-to-use at-home rituals that you and your lover can try are explored in Chapter 6. They range from a blissful water and salt exfoliation bath to making matching magic amulet bags.

Chapter 7 explores the orgasmic "apparatus" of your body and shows you how to enjoy sex on your own, how to find the male or female G-spot, and how to enjoy sexual relations into the golden years of 60 and beyond.

Many of the ideas and techniques you will find in *The Natural Guide to Great Sex* may take you into new territory. To insure your own and your partner's safety, consult a qualified health care professional before making radical adjustments to your behavior.

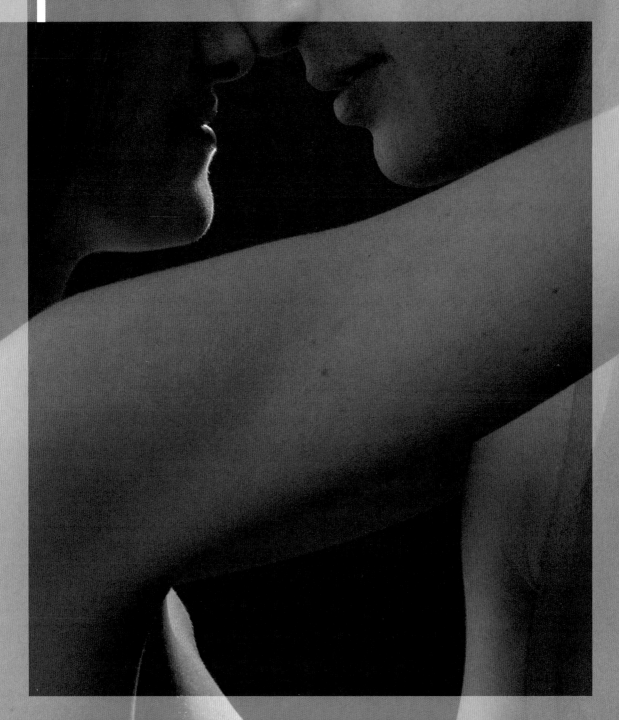

Hormones are complex compounds manufactured within the body. They act as a telegraph feedback system, triggering organs either to activate or turn off. As you will discover in this chapter, both men and women have the same sex hormones, although they are present in different ratios and may act in different capacities in each gender. Here you will learn how to balance and support sex hormone production and function to maximize the health benefits associated with adequate hormone levels.

The Hormone—Sex Connection

Hormones are chemical messengers that circulate through the body, acting like the individual notes that combine to compose a symphony. Musically, when each note is played correctly in terms of tone and amplitude, a harmonic resonance is created that results in a soothing and rewarding vibratory pattern. However, if any player is off-key, the result can be a disturbing dissonance. Likewise, each hormone in the body is dependent on the others. They are all linked in a perpetual feedback loop that influences the fluid movement of each of the other hormones.

Hormones also affect the function of all metabolic processes, including sexual function. All of the sex hormones are important in both men and women, although some of them are more often associated with one sex. For instance, *follicle stimulating hormone* (FSH) is involved in the development and release of the egg in women, but is also needed for sperm production in men. *Luteinizing hormone* (LH) influences the formation of the *corpus luteum*, or yellow body, which releases progesterone in women and also stimulates the production of testosterone in men.

Estrogen:
The Feminine Hormone

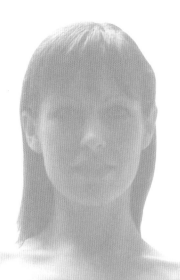

Estrogen is not just one hormone, but a group of hormones that act together as a controlling force in the development of female characteristics (such as breasts) and are vital to all aspects of sexuality and fertility. The three main varieties of estrogen are estrone (E-1), estradiol (E-2), and estriol (E-3). Conventional physicians will usually test only for estradiol, while holistic healthcare practitioners will monitor levels of all three. In addition to the ovaries of women, estrogen is produced in the adrenal glands of both sexes, as well as in the testes of men. Estrogen levels change constantly throughout the monthly menstrual cycle in women and tend to decrease with age.

ESTROGEN AND HEALTH

The balance of the various types of estrogen will either help or hinder health. For instance, aggressive estrogens can cause health disturbances ranging from mild annoyances (such as breast tenderness) to illnesses as serious as cancer in both men and women. Aggressive estrogens can be tempered, or opposed, by milder estrogens. More aggressive estrogen levels are caused by a diet high in pesticides, herbicides, and toxic chemicals, as well as by toxic emotional states. Milder, protective estrogens are encouraged by a low stress level and a healthy diet.

High estradiol levels in men have been linked to irritability, depression, and sexual dysfunction. Low estrogen levels develop in menopausal women. Hormone replacement therapy (HRT) is often recommended by doctors to offset the associated symptoms, including vaginal dryness and loss of sex drive. However, due to the serious adverse effects of pharmaceutical HRT, many women are choosing more natural options for increasing estrogens. These options include the use of foods (pomegranate, green beans), herbs (black cohosh, dong quai, red raspberry), and exercise (yoga postures, such as the shoulder stand).

In order to help balance your own estrogen levels, you have a number of options:

- Consider consulting a holistic healthcare practitioner to test you for all three types of estrogen, and progesterone, testosterone, and dehydroepiandrosterone (DHEA).[1]
- Consider natural alternatives to conventional HRT, including the foods and herbs mentioned above.
- Consider adding exercise to your daily routine, such as yoga, walking, dancing, or swimming. It is always best to choose something you really enjoy so you will keep it up.
- Consider the use of bioidentical hormone therapy (which must be prescribed by a physician), as discussed later in this chapter.

Testosterone:
The Libido Hormone

Testosterone is responsible for the development of male traits, such as facial hair and a deep voice. However, testosterone is vitally important to both men and women. Testosterone is produced in both sexes in the adrenal glands and liver. Women's ovaries produce a small amount, while the testes in men are the highest testosterone producers.

Testosterone is the main hormone responsible for feelings of lust in both sexes. Holistic health practitioners regularly monitor the level of free testosterone, which is most accurately determined by saliva testing. In the blood, sex hormone binding globulin (SHBG) binds a high percentage of the available testosterone. This renders it unavailable to perform functions such as increasing sex drive. Testosterone can also adhere to binding sites on cell membranes within the brain.

The differences between men and women in the sites where testosterone can bind tells us a lot about the mind–body connection that is so much a part of sexuality. For instance, testosterone fits into receptor sites in the area of the brain in men that relates to immediate lust, while the same hormone fits into receptor sites in the female brain that are associated with emotional attachment. What a clear case of science lending credence to commonly observed behavior! If testosterone levels are found to be low, along with symptoms of a decreased sex drive, testosterone replacement therapy can be a great remedy.

RAISING TESTOSTERONE LEVELS

Many herbs have been proven to increase testosterone levels, such as ginseng, damiana, muira puama, epimedium (horny goat weed), sarsaparilla, wolfberry, and yohimbe. (These herbs are discussed in detail in Chapter 2.) Prescription drugs are available that can deliver testosterone to the body by rubbing it on the skin. This medication is well tolerated, and can be used by both men and women to help raise testosterone levels. Just as there are several different forms of estrogen, the same is true for testosterone. Dihydro testosterone, or DHT, is often referred to as "bad testosterone" and is linked to enlarged prostate and male pattern baldness.

Here are some options that can help you manage your own testosterone levels:

- Have your testosterone level tested to see if supplementation should be considered.
- Monitor your levels of DHT, since high levels may lead to prostate problems.
- Take occasional supplements of ginseng and other herbs if needed.

DHEA
(Dehydroepiandrosterone)

DHEA is a compound that can be thought of as androgenous because it is a precursor to both male and female hormones. DHEA levels are high in the teens and early twenties, then decrease with age. Scientific research has suggested that DHEA may have powers that could be called miraculous, especially in the area of sexual health. For example, one study showed that postmenopausal women experienced improved sexual arousal with DHEA supplementation.[2]

DHEA has been hailed as an antiaging nutrient, proving its usefulness for enhanced energy, accelerated sex drive in men and women, improved sleep, happier mood, and reduced stress. However, before you run out and start popping over-the-counter DHEA capsules, I suggest you do the following:

- Have your DHEA level measured through a saliva test. If a person's level is too high, it can cause side effects such as facial hair growth in women, and acne, insomnia, and irritability in both sexes.[3]
- If you need to raise your DHEA levels, you can do so through exercise, proper diet, and stress reduction.
- You can also raise DHEA levels through the specific energy-work technique described in Chapter 3. For example, yoga can help to stimulate the adrenal gland's ability to make DHEA. Increasing consumption of food rich in essential fatty acids, such as wild salmon, can give your body the nutrients necessary to enhance DHEA.

Stimulating the Ring of Fire

C. Norman Shealy, M.D., Ph.D., was the first person to describe the technique of Stimulating the Ring of Fire. Dr. Shealy found through research that people can increase their DHEA levels, and therefore rejuvenate their sex lives, by stimulating particular acupuncture points.

The Ring of Fire connects the "battery points" of the body. It establishes an energetic feedback loop between the all-important pineal gland, pituitary gland, heart, autonomic and sympathetic nervous systems, thyroid gland, adrenal glands, testicles/ovaries, and uterus/prostate. When these glandular energy centers of the body are communicating harmoniously, a feeling of vibrancy and health is the happy result.

The following acupuncture points can be stimulated by several means. The simplest way is to apply finger pressure in a circular motion on each point. Dr. Shealy also recommends the use of a specialized electronic TENS device (a medical device that sends a mild electronic signal through the skin), which can be used to stimulate the points.

POINTS TO STIMULATE THE RING OF FIRE

To stimulate your own Ring of Fire, follow these steps:
- See the illustration (right) to help locate the points.
- Begin with GV 20: the center of the top of the head.

Apply finger pressure in a circular motion. Please note that when pressure is placed on the point it may be tender.

- Rub progesterone cream on the point to enhance the production of DHEA. Repeat these steps for each of the following points:

LI 18: the sides of the neck, just below the skull

MH (Triple Burner) 6: measure one inch (2.5 cm) above the center of the front of the wrist

CV 18: a slight indentation on the midline below the bone across the bottom of the neck

B 22: one inch (2.5 cm) on each side of the spine at the second lumbar vertebra

CV 6: one inch (2.5 cm) below the belly button

CV 1: the point on the midline of the underside of the perineum, between the anus and the genitals

K 3: in the hollow on the inside of each ankle

Below: The Ring of Fire acupuncture points.

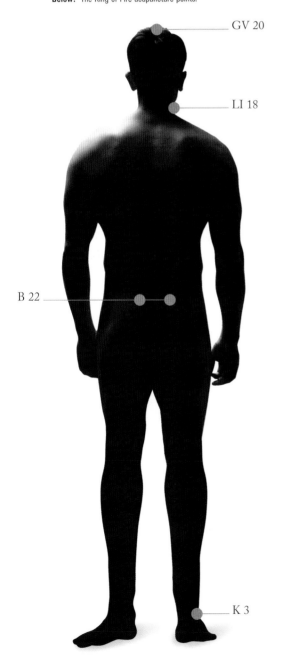

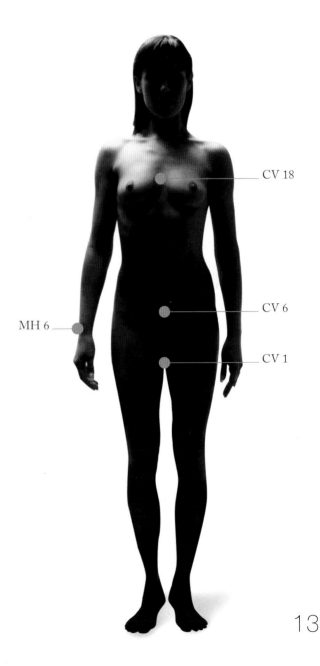

GV 20

LI 18

B 22

K 3

CV 18

MH 6

CV 6

CV 1

Progesterone:
The "Happy Mood" Hormone

Progesterone is intricately connected to sexual function. Although its role may be better defined in women, it is equally important in men. The word *progesterone* is from the Latin *progestin*, which means "before pregnancy," because of its role in preparing the body for pregnancy.

The beneficial effects of natural progesterone include reduction of blood clotting and water retention, promotion of healthy cell division, and mood balancing. Men require sufficient progesterone for testosterone production. Progesterone also helps prevent "good testosterone" from converting to DHT ("bad testosterone"). Progesterone levels may be enhanced by natural supplements such as magnesium, chastetree berry (vitex agnus-castus), licorice root, and wild yam.

Here are some things you should keep in mind about progesterone:

- You can have your progesterone level measured by saliva testing.
- You can apply progesterone in the form of a topical cream, which has a molecular structure identical to natural progesterone. The cream is rubbed directly onto the skin. This cream is easily absorbed and is a wonderful aid to both sexes for revving up progesterone-related sexual wellness.

If you need long-term progesterone replacement, it is best to get a prescription for oral natural progesterone because, over time, the cream may cause a buildup of progesterone in the tissues and lead to an overabundance of progesterone.

Remember that natural progesterone is not medroxyprogesterone, which is an artificial compound with a long list of adverse effects.

OXYTOCIN: THE ORGASMIC CHEMICAL

Oxytocin is a chemical that causes muscles to contract in a rhythmic wave. It is involved in creating the pulsing delight of orgasm in both men and women,[4] and is also involved in contractions during childbirth. At high levels it lowers blood pressure and elevates feelings of well-being.

Right: Natural progesterone has a mood balancing effect.

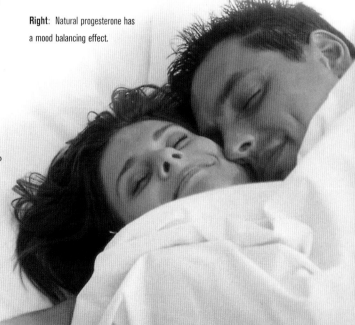

Bioidentical
Hormones

In addition to having a healthy diet, exercising daily, following stress reduction techniques, and using the herbs and supplements discussed in this book, one of the most remarkable antiaging therapies available is the use of pharmaceutical-grade natural hormones, referred to as "bioidentical hormones." These hormones are quite different from the kinds of hormones that have been used for conventional hormone replacement therapy (HRT) for both men and women, and which have molecular shapes that vary greatly from those that the human body manufactures. In contrast, bioidentical hormones have the same shape as naturally occurring hormones.

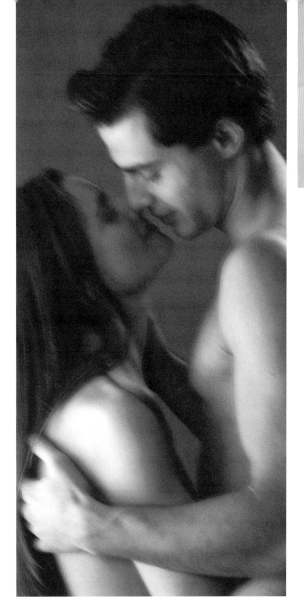

Above: Bioidentical hormones can be effective antiaging agents.

SALIVA TESTING

In order to discover which bioidentical hormones to prescribe for a particular person, holistic doctors choose to use saliva testing to determine an individual's hormone level. While conventional physicians use blood testing, it is not as useful as saliva testing, because most of the hormones that circulate in the blood are bound to carrier proteins and are not available to bind to target tissues. The hormones that have been studied most extensively in saliva include estrogens (estradiol, estrone, and estriol), progesterone, testosterone, and DHEA.

When you have a saliva test done to determine your own hormone level, I suggest the following:

- After getting your results, ask your physician to prescribe an individualized hormone complex based on your exact results. This is again different from conventional HRT, where everyone is given the same prescription.
- Have the prescription filled by a compounding pharmacy.
- Either administer the hormones orally via a capsule or externally as a cream that you rub on the skin.

Saliva testing is really a simple procedure, but the results are well worth knowing.

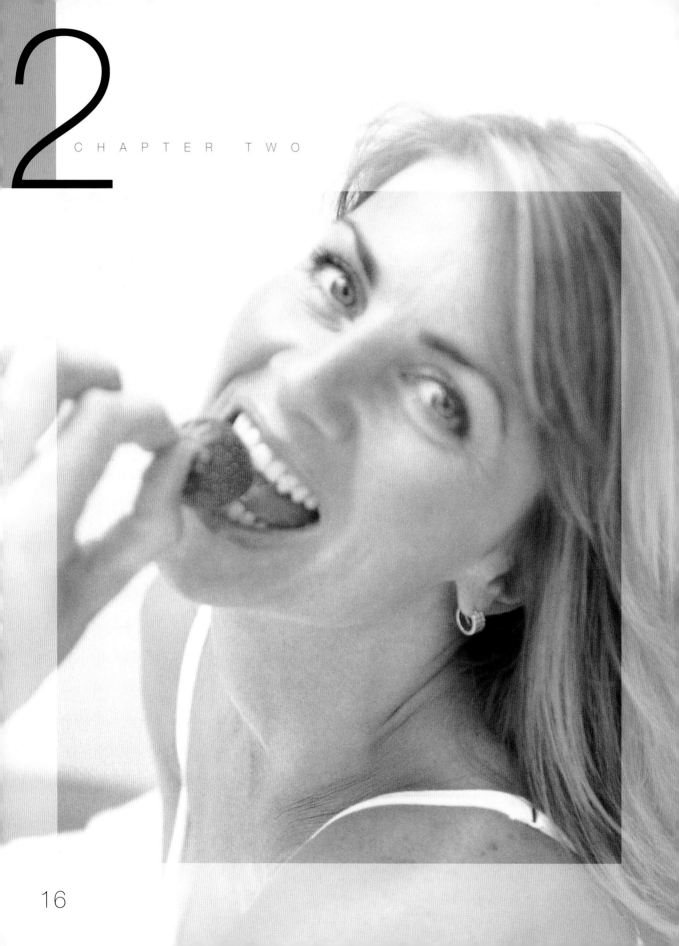

2

In this chapter, you will discover the many avenues that can be opened through aphrodisiacs to enhance sex. Foods, herbs, and vitamins/nutrients can be safely and effectively used as libido boosters. Some of these substances have undergone scientific scrutiny and the mechanisms of their enhancing abilities are now understood. Others have stood the test of time afforded by longtime traditional use.

Natural Aphrodisiacs for Men and Women

The term *aphrodisiac* means "something that arouses or intensifies sexual desire." The word probably originated in the early eighteenth century, gleaned from the Greek word *aphrodisiakos*, meaning "arousing sexual desire," and from Aphrodite, the goddess of sexual love.

Humankind's quest for substances that increase both the pleasure and potency of sexual encounters spans the ages. In civilizations past and present, high honors and awards have been given to healers (as well as drug companies) who have been able to produce effective sexual stimulants. Tribal medicine men and women would frequently experiment with plants, gemstones, and animal parts in search of potency elixirs. Cave drawings and ancient manuscripts describe all manner of herbs, teas, and potions that have been used for their true or imagined erotic enhancement potential.

Aphrodisiacs work in several ways. They may directly increase the physical desire to have sex, stimulate the strength and endurance of an erection in men, or increase lubrication and genital sensitivity in women. Very few substances are scientifically proven to do all this on a consistent basis. Most supposed aphrodisiacs act as tonics that increase virility over time, usually by supplying nutrients that feed the glands and organs. Others may relate more to psychological and mind/body interactions.

Foods

Consider the following authoritative comment from the *Encyclopedia Britannica* in reference to the sexually stimulating nature of food:

. . . The combination of various sensuous reactions— the visual satisfaction of the sight of appetizing food, the olfactory stimulation of their pleasing smells, and the tactile gratification afforded the oral mechanism by rich, savory dishes—tend to bring on a state of general euphoria conducive to sexual expression.

A wide variety of foods have been used for their aphrodisiac properties. People often viewed the "seed quality" of foods such as eggs or bulbs to be indicative of their highly sexual nature. Food with a natural phallic shape, such as carrots or asparagus, were also thought to have enhancement value. It is interesting to note that many foods thought to be aphrodisiacs by the ancients are high in nutrients that are needed for successful sexual function, and they prove to be especially effective if a person is low in those nutrients.

Unfortunately, the standard Western diet consisting of highly processed junk food is linked to obesity and almost every degenerative illness known. The same nutrient-rich, naturally based diet that protects the body from the ravages of disease will also enhance the function of all the glands and ensure the production of adequate hormone levels to maintain sexuality into advanced age. The fact is that people who exercise daily, eat a diet high

in organic vegetables, and include foods rich in Omega-3 oils and other essential fatty acids such as nuts and seeds are the most likely candidates to experience a longer, healthier sex life. (Keep in mind that the terms *appetite* and *hunger* are used to describe the desire for both food and sex.)

The following sections describe a number of foods that have gained a reputation as sexual enhancers:

Fruit

AVOCADO

Just picture a large, ripe, green avocado and you can imagine why the Aztecs called the avocado tree *ahuacuati*, which means "testicle tree." Avocados are a great source of the good oils needed for the production of sex hormones.

BANANA

Bananas are one of the most outwardly phallic fruits. Those who have visited the Caribbean may have seen that the flower on a banana tree also has a very strong sexual overtone. Bananas are high in potassium and other vitamins and minerals used by the body to build sex hormones.

BERRIES

Sweet, juicy strawberries and raspberries are often associated with ripe sexuality. Berries are actually the sexual expression of plants because they are the seeds

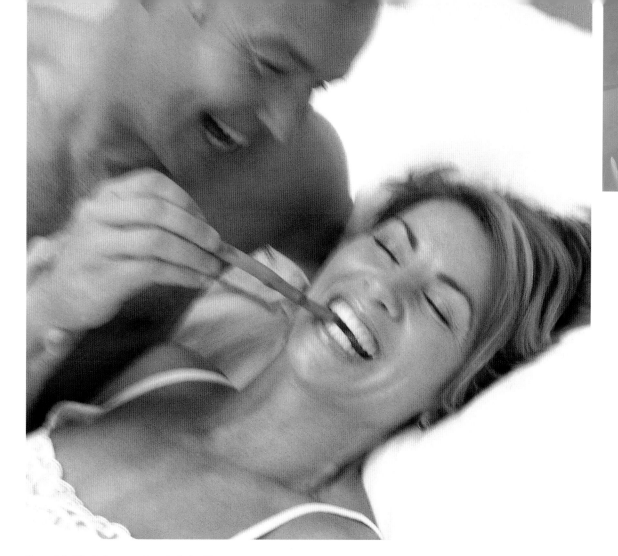

Above: Full of Vitamin E, asparagus is a natural aphrodisiac.

containing fruits. Berries are a perfect lovemaking food, and can be erotically hand-fed to a lover. Berries are high in bioflavonoids and Vitamin C, which heighten health, energy, and sex drive.

FIGS

The fig has a soft quality that has been likened to the female sex organ. Figs are high in Vitamin A, potassium, and calcium, and boast the highest mineral content of all common fruits. Research performed by Rutgers University in New Jersey has determined that dried figs contain Omega-3 and Omega-6 essential fatty acids, as well as a number of phytosterols, which are needed by the body for sex hormone production.

PINEAPPLE

The flamboyant pineapple has been used as a symbol for opulence and glamor for centuries. It often graced bedposts as a decorative addition to "juice up" the marriage bed. Pineapple juice is believed to sweeten seminal fluids, and is included as a treatment for impotence in homeopathic medicine.

POMEGRANATE

The pomegranate has been called the "Love Apple" and has a long history as a sexual symbol. The goddess of love, Aphrodite, supposedly planted it on Cyprus as a gift to lovers. When cut open, it resembles an ovary full of seeds, and has been eaten by both sexes to enhance fertility. In addition to high levels of Vitamin C and potassium, pomegranates contain a form of estrogen called estrone.

Nuts

ALMOND

The aroma of almond has been used to heat up the bedchamber in many societies. Almond paste (marzipan) can be used as a lickable love potion when rubbed onto erotic areas. Licking it off gives pleasure to both parties, as well as enhancing the level of sex-healthy nutrients such as magnesium and Omega-3 fatty acids.

PINE NUTS

Pine nuts have been employed since medieval times as a libido stimulant, as described in the medieval medical manuscript, *Tacuinum Sanitatis in Medicina*. The Greek physician Galen wrote in the second century C.E. that a mixture of honey, almonds, and pine nuts eaten before bed for three nights will increase a man's virility. The Roman poet Ovid includes pine nuts in his poem *Ars Amatoria* ("*The Art of Love*"). Pine nuts are also called pignoli nuts and are often used in pesto recipes. They are very high in zinc, the "love mineral".

Spices

ANISE

Anise is a licorice-scented spice with a seed pod that is in the perfect shape of a star. The Greeks and Romans used it as an aphrodisiac by sucking on the seeds directly or brewing them as a tea.

CARDAMOM

Cardamom is an Indian spice used to help circulation and blood flow to all areas of the body, including the genitals. One ancient remedy for impotence is a drink prepared by gently boiling three cardamom pods in one cup of milk for five minutes. Add one teaspoon of honey.

CAYENNE

A constituent known as *capsaicin* stimulates nerve endings and adds to the heat for which cayenne is well known. It raises the pulse and increases circulation to all areas of the body, including the genitals.

CINNAMON

The distinctive aroma of cinnamon can evoke a strong romantic response in both men and women. Cinnamon helps to balance blood sugar and aids in the maintenance of high levels of energy. Both its scent and flavor help to set a romantic mood.

CLOVES

Cloves have a long history of medicinal use and remain an herbal analgesic treatment for toothaches to this day. Cloves contain chemical constituents that cause a pleasant numbing of nerve endings, and have been used as an aphrodisiac spice in China since the third century B.C.E. In the Netherlands, several medieval herbalists touted the sexual powers of cloves, indicating that drinking clove tea along with milk will make a man desire his woman.

GINGER

The hot, spicy taste of ginger is a stimulant for circulation to all the organs, and has anti-inflammatory qualities that can soothe aches and pains that may get in the way of sexual enjoyment. Ginger can be made into a tea for drinking or used as a hot compress on achy areas of the body. It can really "spice up" your love life.

NUTMEG

Nutmeg can be a dangerous hallucinogen if used in large quantities, but it is a sexy spice when sprinkled with a light touch. It was used by Arabs, Greeks, Romans, and Hindus for its sexual effects, and was prized by Asian women for this purpose. Nutmeg contains myristicin, a chemical similar to the hallucinogen mescalin. One recipe calls for crushing a boiled egg along with honey and nutmeg, and eating it one half-hour before making love to sustain an orgasmic state.

Vegetables

ARUGULA

The bitter taste of arugula releases digestive enzymes that allow the body to absorb the micronutrients needed for sexual health. This vegetable has been touted for its aphrodisiac properties since the first century C.E. Grind arugula into a paste with pine nuts, pistachios, and basil for a love-enhancing pesto sauce.

ASPARAGUS

Asparagus is obviously a phallic food, with a clear representation of both the shaft and the head of a penis. Practitioners of traditional Chinese medicine considered asparagus to be a food that dispels anger. Steam asparagus and share a shaft with your lover. Its rich Vitamin E content is also sex healthy!

CARROT

The phallic-shaped carrot has a long history of use as a natural sex toy and can still be enjoyed in this manner. Carrots are highly nutritious and are full of mixed carotenoids that are needed for sex gland health.

CILANTRO

This dark green vegetable produces the seed called coriander that is used as a spice. Both coriander and cilantro have been used for their aphrodisiac qualities for at least a thousand years. Cilantro was mentioned in *The Arabian Nights*. Cilantro is high in vitamins and minerals.

FENNEL

The licorice flavor and bulbous nature of fennel, along with the elongated stalk, have sustained its use as an erotic vegetable since ancient Egyptian times. In the 1930s, scientists considered using fennel as a source of estrogen because it contains estragole, an estrogenlike substance. Research has proven its libido-enhancing effect in rats, and fennel is believed to sustain erections and prolong sexual activity.

GARLIC

Although the odor of garlic on a lover's breath may be considered a turnoff, this problem is alleviated if both partners partake. Garlic has traditionally been used in civilizations worldwide for its health-enhancing properties. Modern science confirms its benefits for cardiovascular wellness. Indian spiritual traditions insist that yogis who wish to be celibate refrain from consuming garlic because it increases "heat" to the genital areas.

Other Foods

ASAFETIDA

Asafetida is prepared from a plant with the exotic name of "devil's dung," which probably refers to the strange odor (from the Latin *foetidus* for "stinking") and strong, garlicky taste of this Indian herb. It has been used to relieve digestive disorders, and as a mild laxative and sexual stimulant in Ayurvedic medicine (from India) for centuries.

BEE POLLEN

This bee product is actually the male sex cell of flowers collected by bees and then used to pollinate the female flower parts. Bee pollen is extremely high in nutrition, and is truly an antiaging superfood with more than 185 nutrients. It increases overall, as well as sexual, energy. Try a small amount at first. People with pollen allergies may be sensitive to bee pollen.

CHOCOLATE

Chocolate is the treat most often associated with love and romance. Its rich, sensuous nature and "melt in your mouth" texture is one of life's pleasures. It has been used by ancient civilizations such as the Aztecs, who called it "food of the Gods." Chocolate is high in magnesium and other minerals. It also contains a compound called phenylethylamine, the feel-good "love chemical," which is found in high levels in people who are in love or experiencing the afterglow that follows orgasm.

COFFEE

The rich, warm flavor of coffee is a hedonistic delight, especially when it is enhanced with exotic additives such as hazelnut and vanilla. Coffee contains caffeine, a stimulant that can add an exciting energy to a nighttime sex romp. (Too much, though, can wear out the adrenal glands and inhibit sex drive.)

EGGS

Eggs were believed to help alleviate most sexual ailments in countries as diverse as Egypt and China, as well as on the continent of Europe. The egg is a natural sex aid on many levels. Obviously it is, in itself, a sex cell that harbors the beginning of life. Egg-shaped stones are used in Oriental traditions to exercise the sexual organs (see Chapter 4). Eggs are high in complete protein, Vitamins A and B_{12}, and most of the minerals required by the body such as iodine, phosphorus, zinc, and selenium.

HONEY

The thick, sticky texture of honey is a seducer's delight. Honey has been used since ancient Egyptian times to remedy impotence. The term "honeymoon" refers to the use of mead, a fermented drink made from honey, by both partners on the first night of their marriage to relieve first-time anxiety and begin nuptial bliss on a sweet note.

LICORICE

Licorice root provides a uniquely sweet, sensuous flavor. It has long been favored in traditional folklore for its love- and lust-enhancing properties. Licorice candy is flavored with anise, not true licorice, in the United States. Licorice root contains compounds needed for the formation of female sex hormones and also supports the adrenal glands (in men and women), which are important for strength, energy, and sexual stamina. The Smell and Taste Foundation in Chicago has discovered that women find the smell of licorice an erotic stimulant.

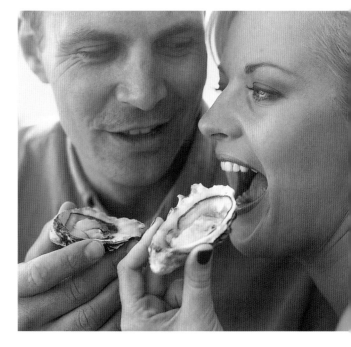

Above: Eating raw oysters can be a sensuous treat.

OYSTER

Oysters enjoy a long history as an aphrodisiac. Aphrodite, the Greek goddess of love, is often pictured rising out of the sea on an oyster shell. Romans documented the oyster as an aphrodisiac, especially since it was considered to look like female genitalia. Oysters are high in protein and minerals such as iodine, phosphorus, and zinc. Zinc is particularly important because it is linked to testosterone and sperm production, as well as to vaginal lubrication.

VANILLA

The long vanilla bean is suggestive of a phallic shape, while the name of this lush flavoring spice is derived from the same root word as "vagina." The bean is the dried fruit of the orchid *Vanilla planifolia*, which also visually mirrors female genitalia. The warm, rich scent and taste of vanilla is associated with love and lust. The medical book *Swedish Pharmacopoedia* (1849) recommended vanilla as an aphrodisiac acting through its odor as much as through its taste.

Recipes
For Lovers

Here are a few recipes that have had tried-and-true success with lovers. Remember that the mood and mode are just as important as the ingredients. As you prepare the meal, visualize the intended outcome. Infuse the ingredients with the intention of your desire. You will not be disappointed!

Fennel, Pineapple, Pomegranate, and Pine Nut Salad

Ingredients

1 fennel bunch, thinly sliced stalks and bulb
1 orange, sliced into wedges (skin removed)
1 whole pomegranate
20 pine nuts
15 mint leaves

1 In a medium-size salad bowl, combine sliced fennel and orange wedges.

2 Scoop all the red seed pods out of the pomegranate and mix them with the fennel and orange slices.

3 Sprinkle the pine nuts and mint leaves on top of the mixture.

4 Serve within one hour of preparation. (You will need an extra bowl to spit out the pomegranate seeds, after sucking off the red juice.)

Oysters on the Half-Shell

1 Split some raw oysters on a decorative plate.

2 Have sliced lemons, limes, and cayenne hot sauce available.

3 Feed each other the slippery oysters.

Aphrodisiac Smoothie

Ingredients

1 cup organic vanilla soy milk or rice milk
2 cloves
1 cardamom pod
1 cinnamon stick
1 banana
2 ice cubes
½ cup organic vanilla yogurt

1 Blend all ingredients in a blender.

2 Share with your lover!

Herbs

Women and men throughout the ages have experimented with various plant substances in an endless search for useful aphrodisiacs. Many folkloric tales of sexual potency are linked to elixirs derived from plants. Although some of these stories are simply "old wives' tales," those old wives may well have held the knowledge that kept them happy and healthy into advanced years. Many herbs have stood the test of time in recognition of their ability to stimulate and sustain sexuality during a particular lovemaking session or over a lifespan into advanced age.

SEX-ENHANCING HERBS

In this section I look at some of the herbs that both ancient shamans and modern scientists credit with the ability to enhance sex. Some of these herbs have been studied by scientists specifically for their ability to increase sexual prowess. Many others have a long history of traditional use, although they have not as yet been put to the test by the gold standard of science. Dosage recommendations are for a normal 150-pound (68-kg) person, and may vary greatly. Cautions reflect specific known health problems that have been associated with a particular herb. If I write "no known adverse effects," it means none are known at the time of writing, but that does not guarantee safety for a given individual. As with all nutritional therapies, do not use any of these while pregnant, nursing, or taking prescription medications, except under the advice of your healthcare practitioner.

DAMIANA

(TURNERA APHRODISIACA, DIFFUSA)

The leaves of the damiana shrub have a long history of use as an herbal medicine in Mexico, dating back to the ancient Aztec and Mayan civilizations. The species name of damiana, *aphrodisiaca*, refers to the best-known use of this herb, which is as an aphrodisiac and sexual stimulant for both sexes. It is also used for its ability to tone the mucous membranes of the reproductive organs.

Along with other chemical constituents, damiana contains betasitosterol, a phytosterol that may be involved with its effects on the sexual organs. As we often see with herbal remedies, age-old folklore traditions are again collaborated by scientific research. Besides its qualities as an aphrodisiac, you'll also find that damiana is a helpful tonic for the nervous system, the genitourinary tract, and the kidneys.

Damiana was listed in the *National Formulary* from 1888 to 1947, and was recommended by physicians for menstrual problems including headache, acne, insufficient flow, delayed menstruation in adolescent girls, irritability, and lack of sexual desire.

In Jamaican folk medicine, it is called *Ram Goat Dash Along*, because when male goats eat it, their libido increases dramatically! Traditionally, shamans have used damiana during rituals because it helped to break inhibitions and promote the feeling of "astral travel" to explore spiritual dimensions.

DOSAGE Tea: Add 1 tsp crushed or powdered leaf to 1 cup hot water. Steep for 10–15 minutes. Drink 2–3 cups/day.

Tincture/Extract: 10–20 drops 3 times/day

Capsules: 300–500 mg 3 times/day

CAUTIONS *No cautions have been noted for the use of this herb, except a slight laxative effect.*

FENUGREEK

(TRIGONELLA FOENUM-GRACEUM)

Fenugreek has been recognized as a medicinal plant for centuries. Egyptians, Greeks, and Romans used the aromatic seeds extensively and harem women used it to increase the size and roundness of their breasts. Today, the herb is often recommended by herbalists to nursing mothers to improve their milk supply.

Mix powdered fenugreek seeds with water or oil to make a soothing paste that can be used as a skin emollient.

Below: Damiana can be used as a sexual stimulant for both sexes.

To use fenugreek as an aphrodisiac, brew some fenugreek tea or take fenugreek capsules or tincture according to the suggested dosage. Taken internally, fenugreek helps to stabilize blood sugar. The rich combination of nutrients in fenugreek includes choline and trimethyamine (a sex hormone in frogs), Vitamins A, B_2, B_6, B_{12}, D, and essential oils.

The aromatic compounds in the fenugreek seeds have a maple syrup sort of odor. Try chewing fenugreek seeds to freshen the breath before a romantic encounter.

DOSAGE Tea: 1 tsp seed in 1 cup hot water. Steep five minutes. Drink 1–3 cups/day

Tincture/Extract: 10 drops 2 times/day

Capsules: 500 mg 2 times/day

Poultice: Soak ground seeds in enough hot water to make a paste. Mix with oil. Apply to skin.

CAUTIONS *No adverse effects are known. However, if too much is used during nursing, the urine of mother and child may start to have a maple syrup odor, and could potentially*

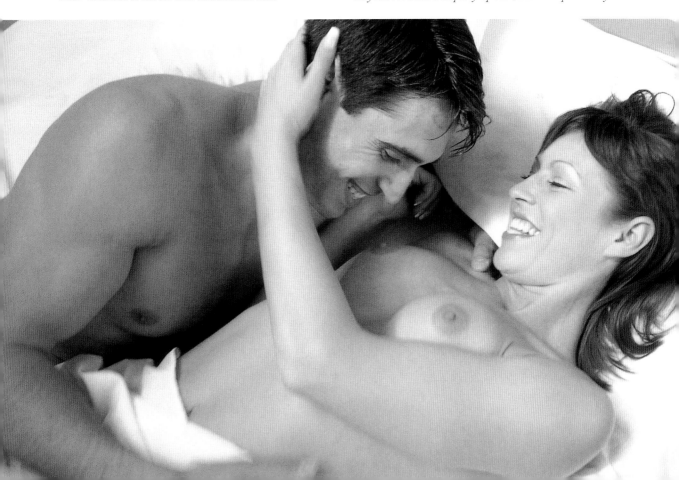

lead to a misdiagnosis of "maple syrup urine disease," a serious genetic abnormality that interferes with the correct metabolism of certain amino acids.

GINSENG *(PANAX GINSENG)*

The name *ginseng* refers to several plant species. The most common species are *Panax ginseng* (called Chinese or Korean ginseng) and *Panax quinquefolia* (American ginseng). The human-shaped root was known as "man with thighs spread apart" by Native Americans.

The Greek word *panacea* is reflected in the name *panax* because of the wide range of healing effects attributed to this root.

Below: Ginseng can help men to maintain erectile function.

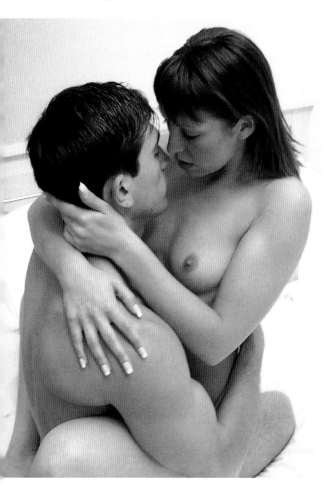

Men who are having erectile problems can benefit from taking Korean red ginseng in the recommended dosage, according to recent studies.[1] Improvements in the ability to achieve and maintain an erection may be experienced. Ginseng confers a youthful vigor to men and women alike for overall as well as sexual health.

DOSAGE Capsules: 500–600 mg/day
CAUTIONS *Ginseng Overuse Syndrome may produce symptoms of insomnia, irritability, anxiety, and heart palpitations, probably due to heightened testosterone levels. These effects are rare, and most often seen in young men using too much ginseng, probably because they already have enough testosterone!*

HORNY GOAT WEED

(EPIMEDIUM GRANDIFLORUM)

According to legend, a goatherd noticed that whenever his goats ate this herb, it revved up their sexual activity tremendously! The Chinese name for epimedium, *Yin Yang Hua*, reflects the effect it has on both women (yin energy) and men (yang energy).

Research suggests that this herb can increase sperm count and semen density in men, and it supports adrenal hormone production in both sexes.[2] It is widely used as an aphrodisiac to increase sexual desire and activity.

If you're feeling run down, take the recommended dosage of horny goat weed in order to improve circulation and boost energy.

DOSAGE Capsules: 500–1000 mg/day
CAUTIONS *No known adverse affects.*

(HO/HE) SHOU WU

(POLYGONUM MULTIFLORUM)

Ho Shou Wu is usually called Fo-Ti in the United States. In China, it is revered for its mysterious properties of rejuvenation and antiaging, and has been used for more than a thousand years as a "royal tonic" that nourishes the blood; cleanses the liver and kidneys; supports the joints, ligaments, tendons, muscles, and sinews; increases the chi energy of the liver and kidneys; and enhances sexuality and fertility in both women and men.

Before you spend money to change your gray hair back to its natural color, consider the following: the name He Shou Wu translates to "Mr. He's Black Hair Tonic," or "King He's White Hair Turned Black." Chinese legends describe a sickly, middle-aged, infertile man named He, who discovered this herb and reversed the aging process. He fathered many children into old age and turned his gray hair back to jet black!

DOSAGE 5–10 pills, 3 times/day

CAUTIONS *May have a slight laxative effect. One case of liver toxicity has been reported.[3]*

KAVA KAVA (PIPER METHYSTICUM)

Kava kava grows in the South Pacific Islands and in Hawaii. It is a wide-leafed vine, relative to the pepper plant. The part of the plant used to make the medicinal extract is the large root, or rhizome. It has been used for thousands of years; indeed Captain Cook described its use in 1768 during one of his South Sea voyages. Today, kava kava is used to relax the body and mind, produce a tranquil state, enhance sociability and friendliness, and ease pain.

Kava kava is touted as an aphrodisiac for women, although it may produce enough muscular relaxation to interfere with an erection in men.

The most common use of kava kava in Western medicine is as an antianxiety agent. The active ingredients in kava kava include kava lactones.

You can find kava kava in health food stores as a prepared extract or capsule, which may be standardized to contain 30 to 50 percent kava lactones. Traditional use of kava kava involves pounding the fresh root into a pulp and then cooking it into a thick tea or soup. It is often served in a coconut shell. However, when prepared in this fashion, the kava drink tastes bitter and causes a tingling sensation on the tongue and throat.

DOSAGE Tea: 2–3 cups/day
Extract: 20 drops
Capsules: 100 mg

CAUTIONS *High doses of kava kava over extended periods of time can cause a rough skin condition called kava dermatitis. It is reversible if kava kava is discontinued. Kava kava can change the way you feel. When first using kava kava do not drive or operate heavy machinery. Try it first in the evening, before a lovemaking session. There are a limited number of cases of liver toxicity that may be linked to kava kava use.*

MUIRA PUAMA (PTYCHOPETALUM OLACOIDES)

Muira puama is known as "Warrior Wood" and "Potency Wood," and is used by the people of the northern Amazon area in Brazil to address many health issues. It is considered a tonic for the neuromuscular system[4] and helps with joint pains, menstrual cramps, PMS symptoms, and mental disturbance. The entire plant is used in medicinal preparations and contains sterols, including betasitosterol, which may account for its activity as a sexual stimulant.

If you are having difficulty achieving an erection, you can try muira puama, which is listed in the British Herbal Pharmacopoeia for the treatment of impotence.

In Brazil, muira puama is used by both men and women to increase libido and sexual performance.

Studies in France have verified its usefulness for men for both increased libido and treatment of impotence. You can find muira puama in health food stores and on-line as both an herbal extract and capsule.

DOSAGE Capsules: 500 mg/day

CAUTIONS *No known adverse effects.*

QUEBRACHO

(ASPIDOSPERMA QUEBRACHO-BLANCO)

Quebracho is an evergreen tree that grows in South America, where it has been used traditionally by native people. It was introduced into Europe as a medicine in 1878. The bark of the tree is the part used as medicine.

You can use quebracho for fevers, blocked circulation, and respiratory problems such as asthma.

Quebracho's influence on improving circulation may be the action that has aphrodisiac properties, as it allows blood to freely flow to the sex organs. Since the tea has a very bitter taste, it may be easier to use quebracho in capsule form.

DOSAGE Fluid extract: 1–2 ml 2 times/day
Capsules: 250 mg 2 times/day
CAUTIONS *No adverse effects known. Quebracho is generally recognized as safe. However, do not use this herb if you tend to have high blood pressure.*

SARSAPARILLA *(SMILAX OFFICINALIS, SPEC.)*

The name sarsaparilla is derived from the Spanish words *sarza* for "bramble" and *parilla* for "vine." During the 1500s, sarsaparilla was used extensively to treat syphilis and other STDs (sexually transmitted diseases). Men who frequented brothels used it to try to avoid catching these illnesses, although the effectiveness of this use is questionable. Sarsaparilla is best known in the United States as the flavoring agent in root beer, although it has been touted for its overall tonic properties for a wide variety of ailments.

You'll find that sarsaparilla is rich in nutrients including calcium, iron, iodine, manganese, potassium, sulfur, and Vitamins B, A, C, and D.

Sarsaparilla contains active constituents that may help to increase hormones including testosterone and progesterone, and it has been attributed with increased virility in men and desire in women.

DOSAGE Tea: 1–2 cups/day
Capsules: 500 mg 2 times/day
CAUTIONS *The* German Commission E *monograph warns that excessive use of sarsaparilla (many times the recommended dosage) may cause stomach and kidney irritation. You should consult your physician if you are taking any prescription medications.*

SAW PALMETTO *(SERENOA REPENS)*

Saw palmetto has been used as a medicinal plant for centuries by the Seminole Indians in Florida and its use can also be traced back to the Mayan civilization. Native people knew that the saw palmetto berries were ripe when they noticed that the local deer and other animals were looking sleek and sassy.

The berries of this dwarf palm tree are high in fatty acid sterols that have been scientifically studied for their positive effect on reducing the size of an enlarged prostate gland, benign prostatic hypertrophy (BPH). This condition is very common in men over the age of fifty.

Saw palmetto berries have also been used to enhance breast size in women. Traditionally, saw palmetto was considered a sexual tonic for both men and women.

DOSAGE One-half cup fresh or dried saw palmetto berries/day
Capsules: 80–320 mg 2 times/day
160 mg (standardized to 80–90 percent fatty acid sterols) 2 times/day is the common dose
CAUTIONS *No adverse effects have been reported. There is some concern that saw palmetto use may interfere with measuring PSA, but this is controversial.*

YOHIMBE *(PAUSINYSTALIA YOHIMBE)*

Yohimbe is derived from the bark of a tall West African evergreen tree. In its native land yohimbe may be made into a tea, smoked, or processed into a powder and sniffed. In the Western world, yohimbine, the primary active constituent of yohimbe, is also available as a prescription drug, yohimbine hydrochloride, used for erectile dysfunction in men. The herbal form can also be used for erectile dysfunction.[5]

Yohimbe increases testosterone blood levels in both men and women, causing enhanced sex drive. Yohimbe also stimulates circulation to the genitals. This is especially helpful for men with decreased penile circulation, and may offset vaginal atrophy in women.

DOSAGE Dosage is important with this herb. A safe amount is 15–30 mg/day. Stick to the label directions on the product you are using.

CAUTIONS *Do not use if kidney or liver disease, high blood pressure, or heart arrhythmias are present. Possible side effects include anxiety, increased blood pressure, and facial hair growth in women. These side effects are infrequent and reversible. It is interesting to note that some people who experience these effects with the herbal extract have no problem taking the prescription drug! The active ingredients in yohimbine can block the action of the drug brimonidine.*

ZALLOUH *(FERULIS HARMONIS)*

Zallouh grows in the Middle East, and is harvested and sold as a plant-based aphrodisiac by the Syrian army.

The root of this plant has been used as an antiaging and sexual enhancer in traditional folk medicine for centuries. In fact, it is thought to have been used in the time of King Solomon. This herb contains ferulic acid and probably works by dilating blood vessels and stimulating circulation.

Zallouh not only aids those who are experiencing low libido, but has also been reported to increase the sex drive in healthy men and women.

Recent clinical trials validate the efficacy of zallouh root as a treatment for erectile dysfunction.

DOSAGE Capsules: 400 mg–800 mg/day

CAUTIONS *May increase blood pressure; causes flushing and headache in some users.*

Below: Yohimbe can help to increase testosterone levels in both men and women.

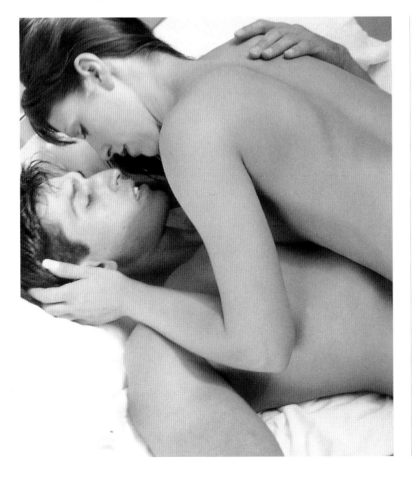

Herbal Aphrodisiac Recipe

Prepare a simple herbal aphrodisiac using the herbs listed below. Purchase liquid extracts, which are available in most health food stores.

Ingredients

Ginseng Extract
Ginger Extract
Oat Extract
Damiana Extract
Muira Puama Extract
Passionflower Extract

1 Combine 20 drops of each herb in one-quarter cup of warm water.

2 Add one-half ounce (15 ml) of amaretto or some other flavored liquor. Relax and enjoy!

Vitamins
Nutrients

Supplements cannot replace a diet high in nutritious foods. Eating a substantial quantity of dark green leafy organic vegetables, whole foods, free-range animal products (in small amounts), and good-quality oils high in Omega-3s is the best way to ensure that the body receives a sufficient level of all the nutrients necessary for optimal health and wellness, as well as vibrant and fulfilling sex.

However, good-quality nutritional supplements, including certain vitamins, minerals, and amino acids, can also be useful. After many years of conventional medicine insisting that supplements are only useful in producing "expensive urine," a study in the *Journal of the American Medical Association* states that "it appears prudent for all adults to take vitamin supplements."[6]

Although there is a plethora of specific nutrients that are essential for many phases of health, the ones mentioned in the sections that follow have specific benefits for sexual function.

ARGININE

Arginine is an amino acid that has many important functions in the body, including the metabolism of protein and formation of nitric oxide. Nitric oxide increases blood flow to the genitals. Additional arginine is required during periods of stress and trauma. Arginine can help decrease LDL ("bad" cholesterol) levels and increase the production of growth hormone. Arginine is also touted as an antiaging factor. This is due to its ability to increase strength and lean muscle mass. It has been shown to increase sperm motility and male fertility.[7]

Arginine, along with yohimbe, has been found to increase sexual arousal of postmenopausal women.[8] You'll find arginine in many readily available food sources: meat, nuts, eggs, coconut milk, and cheese.

B COMPLEX VITAMINS

Vitamin B complex includes a family of eight different vitamins that perform a variety of functions in the body. Many of them moderate the health of the nervous system as well as the growth of different tissues and metabolism of proteins, fats, and carbohydrates. Therefore, the B vitamins as a complex are important in every aspect of health. There are eight members of the B complex family, including B_1 (thiamin), B_2 (riboflavin), B_3, also called B_7 (nicotinic acid, niacin, niacinamide), B_5 (pantothenic acid), B_6 (pyridoxine), B_{12} (cyanocobalamin), folic acid, and biotin. All of the B vitamins are important and work with each other. B_3, B_5, and B_6 are particularly essential for sexual health.

You'll find B complex vitamins in many food sources: chicken, legumes, eggs, green leafy vegetables, and whole grains.

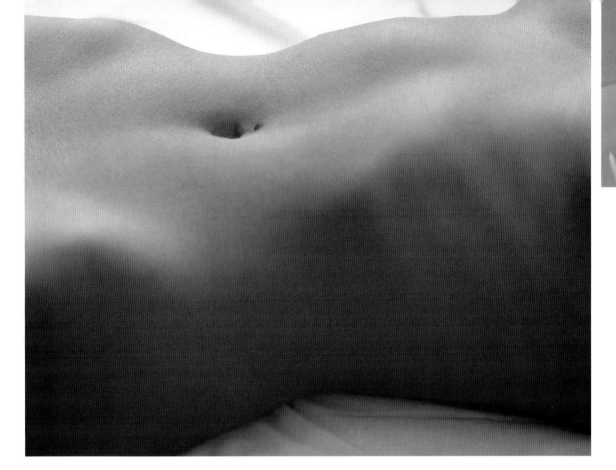

Above: Vitamin A is essential for a smooth, healthy skin.

DOSAGE 50–200 mg/day

CAUTIONS *Vitamin B complex is very widespread in food sources and has not been linked to adverse effects. Some B complex supplements may turn the urine a deep yellow color.*

VITAMIN B$_3$

Vitamin B$_3$ (niacin) is involved in the formation of sex hormones and stabilizes blood sugar. Low levels cause muscle weakness, fatigue, skin sores, irritability, and depression. Antibiotic use or a refined diet high in sugar deplete this nutrient.

Making sure your diet is rich in B$_3$ improves circulation and dilates blood vessels, allowing blood to engorge the sex organs, and increasing lubrication of mucous membranes.

You'll find B$_3$ in many food sources, including meat, chicken, fish, peanuts, brewer's yeast, and wheat germ.

DOSAGE 50 mg/day. Niacin as nicotinic acid may cause a flush, with redness and tingling that lasts about 15 minutes; niacinamide does not cause a flush and may be preferred.

CAUTIONS *Do not take more than 2,000 mg/day. It may cause liver damage.*

VITAMIN B$_5$ *(PANTOTHENIC ACID)*

The name *pantothenic* comes from the Greek word *pantos*, which means "everywhere," because B$_5$ is present in all cells. It assists in the production of adrenal gland hormones, which are important for maintaining energy levels. If your body is low in B$_5$, you can experience generalized fatigue as well as low libido.

Vitamin B$_5$ is widely distributed in food: liver, meat, chicken, whole grains, legumes, broccoli, and cauliflower.

DOSAGE 15–20 mg/day, pantothenic acid, pantothene

CAUTIONS *Loose stools and occasional diarrhea may occur with high doses, but are rarely reported.*

VITAMIN B$_6$ *(PYRIDOXINE)*

Vitamin B$_6$ is intimately connected to the formation of body structures and red blood cells, nervous system function, immune function, and the production of semen and testosterone. B$_6$ is depleted by many factors, including excess protein intake, dyes such as FD&C yellow #5, and several prescription drugs.

Low-grade deficiency is common, especially in people who consume the Standard American Diet (SAD) consisting of highly processed food.

Vitamin B$_6$ is available in food sources such as whole grains, legumes, nuts, and seeds.

DOSAGE Recommended Daily Allowance (RDA): 2 mg/day
Therapeutic dose: 20 mg/day. Pyridoxal 5 phosphate is the most active form, and is preferable over pyridoxine hydrochloride.
CAUTIONS *Occasional side effects have been reported in high doses from 1 g to 6 g. These include neurological symptoms such as tingling in the extremities and interference with muscle coordination.*

VITAMIN C/BIOFLAVONOIDS

Vitamin C functions to repair and maintain healthy connective tissue. It is essential for collagen production, so important for skin and membrane elasticity, including vaginal membranes. Sperm tend to clump together if Vitamin C levels are too low. Vitamin C may help increase the intensity of orgasms. Vitamin C has antioxidant properties and also acts as an anti-inflammatory.

If you have an injury, take some Vitamin C; it helps in tissue repair and reduces bruising and swelling. Bioflavonoids are sister compounds to Vitamin C, and are found along with Vitamin C in many foods. The white pulp under the skin of citrus fruits is high in these nutrients.

You'll find Vitamin C in oranges, grapefruits, kiwis, lemons, rose hips, avocados, parsley, and many other fruits and vegetables.

DOSAGE RDA 60 mg/day. Therapeutic dose: 500 and 5,000 mg/day in divided doses
CAUTIONS *Too much Vitamin C may cause loose bowel movements.*

VITAMIN E

Vitamin E is actually a group of compounds called *tocopherols* (alpha, beta, delta, epsilon, gamma, and zeta). The Greek translation of *tocopherol* is "to bear children," because Vitamin E increases fertility. The main function of Vitamin E is its powerful activity as an antioxidant. It protects all cell membranes from oxidative damage, has proven anticarcinogenic properties, supports cardiovascular wellness, and aids in cellular respiration.

Vitamin E is destroyed by chlorine in drinking water, polyunsaturated fats, and other toxins, so supplementation is recommended.

You'll find Vitamin E in cold pressed oils from sunflower and safflower seeds and almonds, hazelnuts, and wheat germ.

DOSAGE RDA is 200 IU. The therapeutic dose is between 400 and 800 IUs. Check the label; dl-alpha tocopherol is sourced from petroleum distillate and should be avoided. The best form of Vitamin E is mixed tocopherols that include the alpha, beta, and gamma forms, along with tocotrienols.
CAUTIONS *Vitamin E may interact with blood-thinning drugs and enhance their effects. Large doses have been reported to cause headache, fatigue, nausea, double vision, muscular weakness, and gastrointestinal distress.*

Minerals

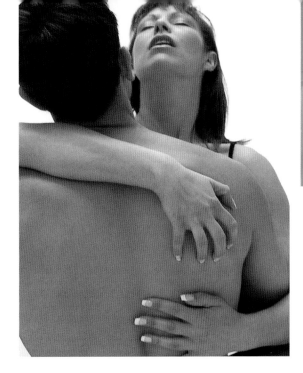

Above: Zinc is essential for healthy nails.

Minerals are essential for health and wellness. They are building blocks for bones, teeth, muscle, blood, nerves, and all cells in the body. They are essential for the flow of information between body systems and are instrumental in the production and function of all the sex hormones. Minerals are widely available in healthy foods, as well as via supplementation.

ZINC

Zinc is a mineral that functions as an antioxidant, an antiviral immune stimulant, and as a component of many enzymes that regulate all metabolic processes in the body. The proper activity of hormones is dependent on adequate zinc levels. High concentrations of zinc are found in seminal fluid and the prostate gland has the highest concentration of zinc of any area of the body. Zinc has earned the title the "love mineral." If you notice white spots under your fingernails, it may be a sign of zinc deficiency. Low zinc levels have been reported in men suffering from impotence and infertility, so it's no surprise that oysters and pumpkin seeds, high in zinc, have been linked to virility in men. Vaginal dryness can also be linked to low zinc levels in women. You'll find zinc in many food sources: whole grains, nuts, seeds, oysters, shellfish, and pumpkin seeds.

DOSAGE 15–50 mg/day. Zinc sulfate is poorly absorbed. Zinc picolinate, citrate, and monomethionine are better absorbed. Read your labels.

CAUTIONS *Prolonged use of more than 150 mg/day can cause anemia, decrease HDL ("good" cholesterol), and decrease immune function.*

MAGNESIUM

Magnesium is a mineral that is often deficient in people who eat the highly processed, refined foods that make up the typical Western diet. Deficiency can cause anxiety, muscle tremors, confusion, irritability, and pain. Cooking and processing depletes magnesium from food. Magnesium helps form bones, activates enzymes, and plays a large part in nerve and muscle function, as well as helping to regulate the acid and alkaline balance in the body. Magnesium can help to elevate the mood and relieve muscle spasms, aches, and pains.

Natural health practitioners often recommend magnesium as an oral supplement or for intravenous infusions. Women have called magnesium intravenous drips "love potions" because they often experience a warm, pulsating sensation in their vaginal area while receiving the magnesium infusions!

Taking 1,000 mg of magnesium one hour before sex can increase the strength of orgasms.

Magnesium is available in many food sources: tofu, nuts and seeds, green leafy vegetables, and seaweed.

DOSAGE 400–1,000 mg, 2 times/day. Magnesium oxide and magnesium chloride are less well absorbed and may have too strong a laxative effect. Magnesium glycinate and magnesium fumerate are better forms for supplementation.

CAUTIONS *Very high doses may cause kidney problems, but this is rare. Loose stools can be controlled by decreasing the amount.*

SELENIUM

Selenium is a trace mineral needed only in small amounts. Selenium works along with Vitamin E in the cell membrane as a powerful antioxidant. Selenium levels are higher in the testes than in other areas of the body. Besides its therapeutic value in reducing inflammation, selenium can also act against the uptake of heavy metals such as aluminum, mercury, and lead, and has helped with depression and fatigue.

Food sources for selenium include liver, meat, and fish. Grains are a good source if the soil where the grains were grown contained a sufficient amount.

DOSAGE 20–100 mcg/day. Avoid sodium selenite. Selenomethionine, extracted from sea vegetables, is better absorbed.

CAUTIONS *High amounts can be toxic and cause hair loss, nail malformations, weakness, and slowed mental function.*

CALCIUM

Calcium is one of the few nutrients that has actually been recognized by the United States Food and Drug Administration (FDA) as having a role in health and disease. Calcium is the most abundant mineral in the body and makes up as much as two percent of total body weight. The main function of calcium is in forming a matrix along with phosphorus that hardens bones and teeth. Calcium is also involved in muscle contraction, nerve function, and heartbeat regulation, and also

moderates the acid/alkaline balance and the way nutrients are taken in and out of the cell across the cell membrane. All of these functions must be working in proper order for optimum sexual function, and especially for orgasms to occur.

Overconsumption of dairy products and other forms of protein causes increased excretion of calcium. Dairy products are also very low in magnesium. Perhaps this is why the United States has the highest incidence of osteoporosis, while countries such as Japan, where very little dairy is consumed, has a low rate.

If you have low calcium levels you may experience anxiety, muscle spasms, leg cramps, and tingling in the extremities. You can alleviate premenstrual syndrome (PMS) symptoms with calcium supplementation.[9]

Food sources for calcium include: dairy products, broccoli, almonds, hazelnuts, oats, lentils, beans, figs, currants, raisins, Brussels sprouts, cauliflower, kelp, and especially kale. Kale is very high in an easily absorbed form of calcium and is an excellent food to include in the diet.

DOSAGE 1,000–1,500 mg. Calcium carbonate is poorly absorbed. Calcium citrate and malate are better choices.

CAUTIONS *People who have a tendency to develop kidney stones should avoid using calcium carbonate.*

IRON

Iron is one of the few minerals that is used in conventional medicine as a supplement. Iron is attached to hemoglobin, the red substance in the blood that carries oxygen to body cells and carbon dioxide back out of the body. Heme iron is the form of iron that is most highly absorbed and is only available from animal sources. This is one reason why vegans often have iron-deficiency anemia.

Iron also functions in DNA synthesis and energy production. If you are low in iron you may experience decreased overall energy, as well as reduced sexual energy.

Food sources for iron include: red meat, organ meat (especially liver), shellfish, and egg yolk. Nonheme iron: oats, millet, parsley, kelp, brewer's yeast, yellowdock root.

DOSAGE 15 mg/day. Avoid ferrous sulfate; it releases a powerful free radical called singlet oxygen (O_1) due to the fentin reaction. Better forms include ferrous fumerate, ferrous gluconate, and ferrous succinate.

CAUTIONS *Iron supplements can cause constipation, black stools, and occasional nausea.*

ESSENTIAL FATTY ACIDS

With the emphasis on "thin is in," the low-fat craze has swept through Western culture like a destructive storm. However, the sad fact is that low-fat diets usually lead to weight gain, since low-fat foods are loaded with sugar or—worse yet—artificial sweeteners such as aspartame. It's important to understand the difference between "good" and "bad" fats.

Fats are part of every cell's phospholipid membrane, which is made up of lipids (in other words, fat) along with phosphorus. The composition, elasticity, flexibility, and strength of these membranes is determined by the kind of fat they contain. Fats found in fast-food French fries, for instance, are hydrogenated and high in transfatty acids. This kind of fat forms a very weak cell membrane that can easily be destroyed by free radicals and other cell-destroying agents, leading to illness and aging. However, if the body has an abundance of healthy fats, strong elastic cell membranes will result.

Essential fatty acids form the sexual lubricating fluids in men and women, and are important in the production of sex hormones. There are several kinds of essential fatty acids that the body cannot make but that must be obtained through the diet. These include Omega-3, -6, and -9 oils. Of these, Omega-3 is often deficient and may need to be supplemented. Another oil that has specific benefits for sexual function is gamma-linolenic acid (GLA).

Food sources for the essential fatty acids include: fatty fish (salmon, halibut, mackerel), purslane (a succulent herb), flaxseeds, flaxseed oil, walnuts, macadamia nuts, GLA-evening primrose oil, black currant seed oil, and hemp seed oil.

DOSAGE Consume approximately 2–3 tablespoons of "good" oils per day. Read individual supplement directions for amount to use.

CAUTIONS *Some people may experience allergic reactions to fish or fish oils, or feel that the supplements "repeat"— the fishy taste of the supplement is experienced after belching. Experiment with different food and supplement sources.*

Below: Calcium hardens teeth for a sexy smile.

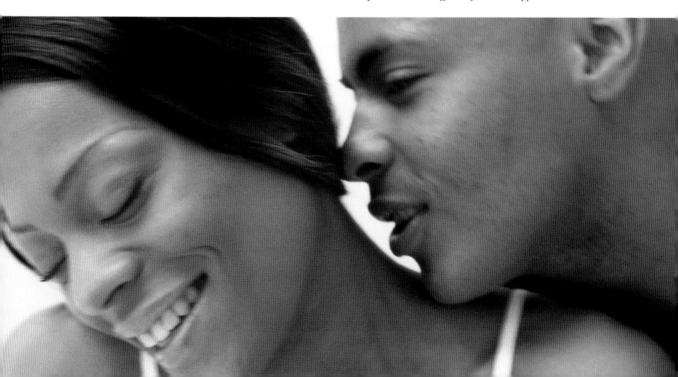

3

In this chapter, we'll investigate exercises used throughout the ages specifically for invigorating the genitals. Some of these systems are from ancient Eastern Taoist, kabbalistic, and yogic practices, which focus on subtle energy manipulations as well as on physical movements and postures. Please note that when engaging in any new exercise or activity or trying a new remedy, it is always best to seek advice from a qualified medical practitioner.

Energy-Based Remedies

Energy-based remedies are not as firmly grounded in the physical realm as are foods, herbs, and nutritional substances. Rather, they work on a more ethereal level. In the case of homeopathic and essence remedies, only the "signature pattern" of the original substance is imparted to the remedy. This is usually done through dilution (adding a miniscule amount of the original substance) and succussion (in the case of homeopathy, a forceful shaking of the remedy followed by banging it against a hard surface, often a holy book) to help the solution memorize the signature pattern.

Although exercise is certainly a physical activity, its benefits broaden to include the energy centers of the body, and are particularly strong when participating in the Eastern Taoist exercises that we explore later in this chapter, along with dance, which enlivens the entire spirit as well as the body.

The physical effects of balanced hormone production and the endorphins (feel-good chemicals) released as a result of exercise are well documented as favorably affecting sexual health. According to research studies, women who exercise regularly tend to have sex more often, get aroused more quickly, and experience satisfying orgasms more often than their sedentary sisters. One study performed on men shows that the frequency of sexual activities, strength of erections, and percentage of fully satisfying orgasms is significantly enhanced in men who exercise.[1]

Of course, the sex act itself is a beneficial form of exercise. It increases the amount of oxygen that bathes the cells, floods the body with endorphins, lowers "bad" cholesterol, and increases estrogen production in women (especially during menopause). Not only that, but the sex act boosts testosterone levels in both men and women, regulates menstrual cycles, increases the production of adrenal hormones, and brings the advantages of aerobic exercise, such as burning calories and fat.

All exercise—such as walking, swimming, or using weights—is good for overall, as well as sexual, health and should be practiced for 30 to 45 minutes per day.

Exercises

Regular exercise is one of the most important things you can do to enhance sexual ability and enjoyment. Exercise strengthens, stretches, tones, increases endurance, and enhances sexual fitness by positively influencing both psychological and physical wellness. Having a positive self-image, along with a dynamic, fit body, increases mental fitness. This creates the "happy self" attitude that is so important to sexual sharing.

Dance

Dance is the most overtly sexual form of exercise. Even a formal dance, such as the minuet, served as a courtship ritual. Dance has been used throughout the ages as a seduction technique as well as a way for couples to gauge how well their bodies move together. In dance, we see the connection between the erotic and divine in the Hindu temple dancers called *Devadis* (servants of the Divine). They fulfilled a dual role of initiating sexual arousal as well as pleasing the gods. Dancing together as a couple can lead to fun and laughter, as well as establishing cosmic harmony.

Try dancing to any music that you enjoy, either alone or with a partner. Dancing while dressed in loose, flowing transparent clothing can lead to a very heated sexual exchange. Many people equate good dancers with proficient lovers and, in fact, that is often the case. Middle Eastern belly dance, tribal African dance, Caribbean

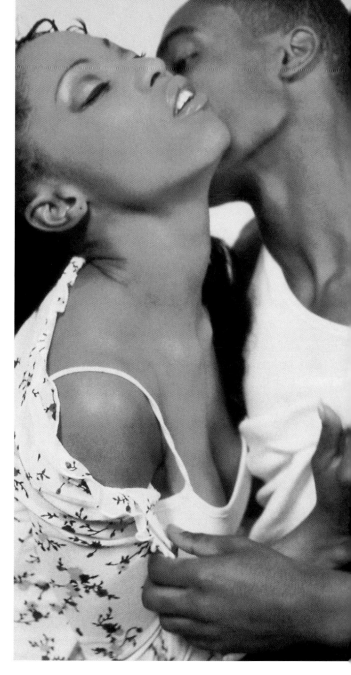

Above: Good dancers are said to make better lovers.

dance, and ballroom Latin dances such as rumbas and mambos emphasize a swiveling of the hips. Learning this movement can help your sex life in many ways. The social exchange afforded by dance may lead you to new partners. In addition, mastering dance hip swivels and applying this movement to lovemaking can send you and your lover to new heights of ecstasy!

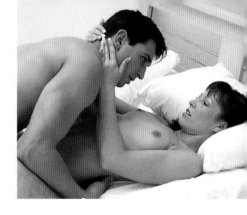

The Kegel Exercise

The Kegel exercise is particularly effective at enhancing the sexual experience for both men and women. The exercise was originally developed by Arnold Kegel, M.D., who originally proposed this method for helping women who suffered from incontinence. This movement strengthens the figure-eight-shaped pubococcygeus (PC) muscle, which supports the sex organs. Without the Kegel exercise, there is very little stimulation to these particular muscles during normal activities, especially since modern lifestyles tend to be sedentary, with hours per day spent on the "derrière."

The conventional way to find the PC muscle is done solo. While urinating, attempt to stop the stream of fluid. Hold for a few seconds, then release and continue urinating. Do this several times. You can also flex this muscle during intercourse. Either of these methods can teach you where the PC muscles are and how to isolate them, so you can do the Kegel.

Incorporate this great sex enhancer in your daily life—not only while having sex or urinating. Squeeze the muscle and hold for two seconds, then release. Repeat five times. Do this two to three times per day. Dr. Kegel originally instructed his patients to practice the move 300 times per day; 100 squeezes at a time, three times per day. You can work up to that if you choose. As you become comfortable, increase the time you hold and add repetitions.

More advanced practice includes clamping the anal sphincter, and adding a "bearing down" movement, all without contracting the buttocks. You can help yourself remember to do the Kegel by coordinating it with other daily activities, such as shaving or brushing your teeth. The time spent commuting to work is ideal. What better way is there to stay stress-free in a traffic jam than to allow your mind to enjoy a sexual fantasy while you Kegel!

1 Isolate the PC muscle. One way to do this is to take a "time out" during face-to-face intercourse. With the penis inside the vagina, the woman attempts to consciously "clamp" her vaginal muscles around the penis.

2 Hold for a few seconds, then release.

3 Repeat a few more times.

4 Now, it's the man's turn. He can "flex" the penis, causing it to move toward the upper wall of the vagina.

5 Hold, release, repeat.

6 This exercise usually feels great to both partners. After trying it one at a time, both partners can clamp and flex simultaneously, and add in synchronized breathing for a beautifully ecstatic moment.

BENEFITS: Increases the flow of blood and nutrients to the pubococcygeus muscle. It also tones and strengthens the muscles and increases elasticity and power.

Hip Rotation

Western cultures tend to emphasize a locked hip, while indigenous cultures worldwide consider free circular motion of the hips to be normal.

You can free up your own hip motions by following these steps:

1 Stand comfortably with your feet shoulder-width apart. It may help to rest your hands on your hips to more easily feel the correct movement.

2 Bend the knees, but remain standing straight.

3 Move your hips around in a circle, first in one direction and then another.

4 Continue for ten rotations in each direction.

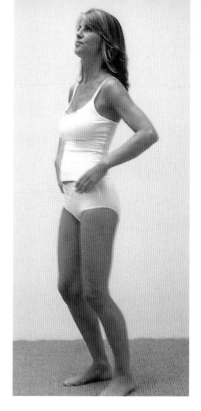

Above: Move your hips in a circle.

BENEFIT: Increases circulation to the sex organs and glands.

The Cat

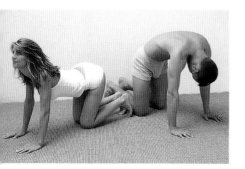

Above: The movements of the Cat can feel sensuous.

There is something about felines that is incredibly sensual. Their soft fur, slow movements, and exotic eyes are alluring. The Cat is an exercise that flexes the whole body and increases circulation along the entire spinal cord:

1 Sit on the floor.

2 Get up onto your hands and knees.

3 Exhale, raising the middle of your back up, while you bend your head to your chest and your lower back toward the floor, like a bow.

4 Reverse, by "bowing" your middle back down, with your head tilted back, and your lower back reaching up. Repeat this up-and-down stretch several times.

5 Once you are comfortable, perform the Cat in a rotation by circling the head and lower back simultaneously, first in one direction, then in the opposite direction.

BENEFIT: Increases flexibility and circulation to the spinal column.

Yoga Exercises

Yoga is an ancient exercise system from India that has become popular with Westerners. The slow, graceful movements of yoga stretch and tone muscles, ligaments, and internal organs. They are designed to increase overall energy within the body by stimulating glands that produce hormones and by bathing cells in oxygen and nutrients.

Regular yoga practice will greatly enhance overall health and wellness, as well as your sex life on many levels. It increases endurance and especially flexibility, allowing for a larger repertoire of sexual positions that you can easily and comfortably accomplish. While the overall practice of yoga is beneficial, there are a few yoga techniques that are especially suited to enhance your sex centers.

Root Lock

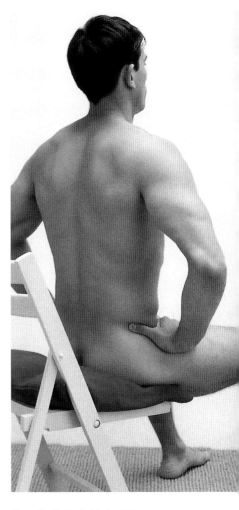

Above: Practice the Root Lock seated.

The Root Lock is similar to the Kegel exercise, but it goes further by incorporating deeper muscles along with breathing techniques:

1 Sit comfortably on a carpeted floor, or on the end of a chair, with feet flat on the floor.

2 Inhale deeply.

3 As you exhale, contract your anal sphincter muscles, your PC muscle (see the Kegel exercise on page 39), and your abdominal muscles, feeling your navel pull toward the back of your spine.

It is normal for the buttocks to contract when you are first practicing this move, but attempt to allow the buttocks to relax.

4 Inhale, release, exhale, engage.

5 Once you are more comfortable, continue to hold the move through several inhale/exhale cycles.

6 To include an energy component to this exercise, focus on accumulating an "energy ball" at the base of the spine. Once you can visualize this swirling ball, allow it to raise up your spine and into the base of your skull.

BENEFITS: Strengthens the PC muscle while incorporating breathing techniques.

Inverted Butterfly

The Inverted Butterfly yoga position opens the heart chakra as well as the pelvis to establish an energy flow between the "love" center and the genitals, energizing your sexual center.

1 Lie on your back and bend the knees, placing your feet flat on the floor.

2 Allow your knees to flare out on each side, as far as they will go. The goal is to touch the knees to the floor. Feel the tension as awareness in your inner thighs.

3 Place both hands lightly under your head and allow the elbows to spread out on either side and touch the floor.

4 Breathe in and visualize yourself as a butterfly with wings outspread. Exhale.

5 Breathe deeply three times and relax into the position as much as possible.

6 Now for the inverted part of this position. Become aware of your genitals. Allow your deep breathing to feel as if you are inhaling and exhaling through your genitals.

7 As you inhale, relax the entire genital area. As you exhale, tense your PC muscles, which surround the genital area.

BENEFIT: Increases circulation to genitals and chest.

Simple Butterfly

This sitting stretch focuses on the inner thighs and opens the genitals, heightening the sensitivity of this area.

1 Sit up straight on the floor. Feel an invisible string starting at your "seat" and coming out of the top of the head.

2 Breathe deeply. Bend both feet, so that they are on the floor.

3 Hold your feet with your hands and place your elbows between your knees.

4 Press your knees toward the floor as far as they will go.

5 Gently bounce the knees up and down.

BENEFIT: Opens hips and pelvis.

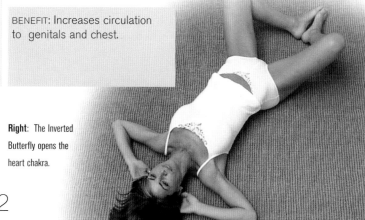

Right: The Inverted Butterfly opens the heart chakra.

Squat (Malasana)

The squat is a position that is common to indigenous people around the world and is the usual position of choice for childbirth.

1 Stand straight and breathe deeply, keeping your feet shoulder-distance apart.

2 Allow your bottom to "melt" toward the floor.

3 Keep the feet flat on the ground for as long as possible.

4 Allow the feet to lift, and relax on the toes while in the squat.

5 Reverse to come up.

BENEFITS: Squeezes and tones all organs in the pelvic area.

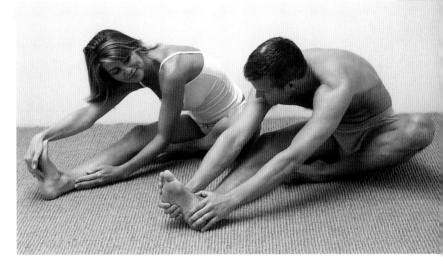

Above: Stretch the leg as far as is comfortable.

Great Seal (Maha Mudra)

Maha means "great" or "large" and *mudra* means "seal" or "body lock." The Great Seal opens the inner thighs and stimulates the genital area.

1 Sit comfortably on the floor.

2 Bring the left heel deeply into the perineum area.

3 Stretch the right leg out at a comfortable angle.

4 Reach down as far as you can and hold your right leg with both hands. The goal is to be able to clasp your right foot.

5 Inhale deeply.

6 Drop your chin to your chest. (This also helps the glands by massaging the thyroid. As the chin presses into the upper chest area, it pushes gently on the thyroid.)

7 Raise the chin and exhale slowly. Release and repeat on the other side by bringing the right heel into the perineum.

BENEFITS: Squeezes the inner thighs; stimulates the genital area.

Taoist Exercises

The term *Tao*, which means "The Way," is used to describe an ancient Oriental spiritual practice. Along with many lifestyle philosophies, the Taoists taught special secret techniques to use sexual energy as a way to increase health and longevity, as well as move toward spiritual fulfillment. The exercise system they devised was guarded as a sublime secret, and taught only through oral tradition to priests and nobility. More recently, however, we have been fortunate to have teachers such as Mantak Chia, who has brought these techniques out of their shrouded past and made them accessible to modern people through the system he calls The Healing Tao. This is a complete and practical system of energy cultivation and development, which leads to the realization of one's boundless self-healing and spiritual potentials.

According to the Taoists, women tend to lose very little *chi* energy (what Taoists believe to be the internal life-force energy) during sex, while men deplete their overall sexual energy when they ejaculate. Therefore, one of the goals for men is to learn to have an orgasm without ejaculation. While many men choose not to take the teaching to this extent, they can still enjoy the benefits of increased health, sensitivity, control, and sexual enjoyment by mastering some of these techniques.

The foundation practices teach one to open and circulate chi through the acupuncture meridians, thereby energizing and harmonizing the body's internal organs and functions. Teachings of the Tao embrace specific techniques as a means of transforming the body. In addition to using controlled sexual positions, a specific dietary regime, exposure of the naked body to natural influences, such as sunlight, and the use of herbal and gemstone remedies, were all prescribed.

The Tao techniques take time to master and are most effective when entered upon with a serious commitment and in-depth study. With that in mind, here are a few Taoist sexual exercises that you can try.

This section contains contributions by Lois Posner, R.N., LMT (see page 124).

Circulating Chi

This technique is basic to the Taoist system and is recommended for both men and women.

Once you master more advanced techniques, you can add the joy of circulating the sexual energy that you harvest from the genitals. This type of energy will feel unique due to its thick, sticky, honeylike quality, which makes it unmistakably identifiable as it creeps slowly up the spine and bathes the brain in its delightful healing nectar.

1 Stand with feet shoulder-width apart, feet strongly connected to the ground, knees slightly bent. (This can also be practiced while sitting on the edge of a chair, with the genitals just forward of the chair edge.)

2 Breathe in and out slowly. Visualize a line that runs all around your body, down the midline, starting at the midpoint of your forehead down the front midline of your torso, to the middle of your pelvis, and then from the front of your body around the perineum to the sacrum in the middle of the

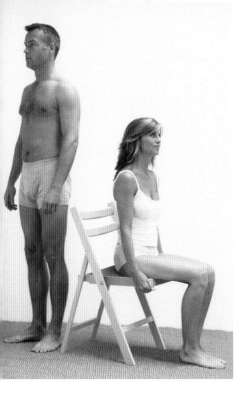

Above: Move your chi by the power of visualization.

Breathing into the Ovaries

This technique for women uses a combination of mind and muscle to extract the life-force energy that lies dormant in the ovaries. Think of the eggs within the ovaries as a source of tremendous potential energy that you can use for your own healing, creativity, and growth rather than just procreation.

lower back. From there the line goes straight up your spinal column to the midline along the back of your skull, back around to your "third eye area" in the midline of the front of your forehead.

3 Visualize the movement of energy through the two main channels of the body, up the back and down the front, while connecting the tongue to the roof of the mouth, on the mound of skin between the two front teeth.

4 Circulate the energy around the circuit 18 times, and then store the energy by allowing it to settle in the navel area.

BENEFIT: Circulates sexual energy, which you can then store for future use.

1 Begin by sitting comfortably on the edge of a chair, feet firmly planted on the floor, shoulder-width apart.

2 Breathe in deeply a few times and visualize the area where the ovaries are located. Gently massage the area while placing your attention deep within it.

3 Very subtly open and close the PC muscles.

4 Visualize the eggs and the entire ovary as glowing and radiating energy.

5 Be aware of any sensation of tingling or warmth in the area.

Now move that energy out toward the midline of the front of your body.

6 From the front midpoint of your body, bring the energy down to where your seat meets the chair—the point between the anus and perineum.

7 Use the Circulating Chi technique to circulate and store the energy.

BENEFIT: Harvests energy from ovaries that you can use for healing and growth.

Egg Exercises

These exercises for women were used in ancient China by queens as well as concubines. Egg exercises can help to maintain youthful sexual vigor well into advanced age. They strengthen the PC muscles, which support the entire pelvic area, and increase circulation of physical fluids (such as lymph) as well as stimulating the more subtle system of energy flow. These exercises act to maintain the core muscles in the lower abdomen and also to seal the lower gate to avoid the leakage of chi energy.

Choose a small- to medium-size, special egg-shaped tool for this exercise. The smaller the egg, the more work your vaginal muscles will have to do. Be sure the egg is smooth, not porous. Take time selecting an egg that has some symbolic significance to you. Obsidian is extremely well suited to use as an egg because its volcanic nature is ideal to enhance the yin or female essence. It is most important to make sure your egg is clean before beginning your exercises.

RULES FOR EGG EXERCISES

- *Always wash your egg with a mild organic cleanser (available in most health food stores) before using.*
- *Boil your "egg" for 20 minutes before you use it for the first time. Always make sure that it has cooled before inserting.*

- *Some people choose to use an organic lubricant, such as sesame or almond oil, for easier insertion into the vagina. It is important not to use any petroleum-based products.*
- *Never practice the egg exercise over tile or cement floors without placing a towel or rug underneath you. This will prevent breakage in case your egg falls out in the event of coughing, sneezing, or unexpected laughter.*

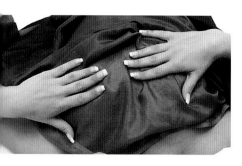

DIRECTIONS FOR EGG EXERCISES

Breast massage precedes the insertion of the egg into the vagina. This activity activates hormone secretions by the breasts and ovaries. Massage both breasts at the same time, gently but firmly. Start at the nipples and work outward in small circles, using a long, smooth silk scarf. Follow with a vaginal massage to stimulate vaginal lubrication.

1 Stand with knees and ankles slightly bent, shoulder-width apart, rooting deeply in order to ground yourself into Mother Earth.

2 Align the spine. Test your spine alignment by standing with your heels several inches away from the wall, with as much of your spine as possible touching the wall, from tailbone to head. Do not strain into the position. It will get easier to straighten as you practice. After aligning, step away from the wall.

3 Take a few deep breaths and relax. Insert the egg completely into the lower part of the vagina.

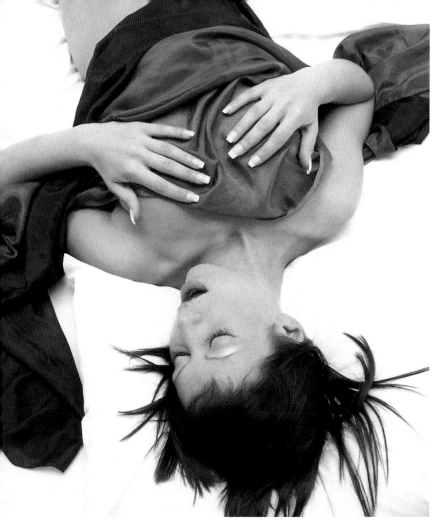

Above: Begin the egg exercise with a sensuous breast massage.

Weight Hanging

Weight hanging is an extension of the Egg Exercise and is also especially good for women. A smooth wooden egg is used because it can be drilled to insert a hook to attach weights.

1 Attach a strong string, dental floss, or fishing line to the hook on the egg.

2 Attach a very small weight to the line. Fishing weights work well because they start out very low and can be increased later on.

3 Follow the instructions as for the egg exercises, except that you "up the ante" to include weights.

4 After weights are attached, they can be gently swung back and forth while you hold the egg firmly in place in the vagina, rather than moving it up and down.

4 Bend your arms at the elbows into a 45-degree angle, with fists gripped slightly in front of you, at hip level.

5 Gently begin to move the egg up and down inside of the vagina, in a controlled wavelike motion. Use the cervix as the top end of the upward wave and make sure to tighten the lower vaginal muscles in order keep the egg securely inside of the vagina. This greatly enhances, strengthens, and increases the control of your inner love muscles, which your partner will surely appreciate!

6 Start out slowly. Keep the egg in for only one or two minutes, and move it up and down only a few times. As you become comfortable with your practice, increase the time up to five minutes or so. The ultimate goal is to no longer have to use the egg, but to be able to consciously move the energy internally with your mind and muscle power.

BENEFITS: Strengthens PC muscles; stimulates subtle energy flow.

CAUTION

Do not try this exercise until you are proficient at egg exercises.

Breathing into the Testicles

This important move for men massages the prostate gland and helps it to maintain the youthful flexibility so commonly lost as men age. According to Taoist teachings, it is important to learn to "lock" this area to prevent the leakage of vital chi energy.

1 Sit up straight on the edge of a chair, allowing your testicles to hang off the edge.

2 Breathe deeply through your nose a few times until you feel relaxed. Visualize your breath going down into the scrotum, filling it with air as if the testes were balloons.

Below: Sit on the edge of a chair for this exercise.

3 Now inhale and slowly draw your testicles up; then exhale and allow the testes to descend.

4 Practice this movement a few times, consciously raising the testicles up and releasing them back down.

5 Practice the "lock" by contracting your anus and PC muscles and then releasing. Once you are comfortable with breathing into the testicles, add the Circulating Chi exercise to move the sexual energy harnessed in the testes up to other organs to energize and strengthen the entire system.

BENEFITS: Massages the prostate; helps maintain flexibility; prevents leakage of energy.

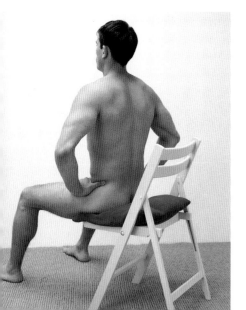

Scrotal Air Compression

Before trying the scrotal air compression exercise for men, practice a downward roll of the abdominal muscles. This movement will be used to force air down into the scrotum. Becoming proficient at scrotal air compression can increase the amount of control men have over sexual arousal. It helps eliminate premature ejaculation, sustains erections for a longer period of time, and allows for more intense orgasms, with or without ejaculation:

1 Sit on the edge of a chair, with testes unsupported.

2 Take a few deep breaths to relax.

3 Keep the tip of the tongue resting on the roof of the mouth. Open the nostrils wide and inhale through the nose, filling the throat with a ball of air.

4 Close off the throat and swallow the ball of air into the chest, below the diaphragm muscle.

5 Use the downward roll of the abdominal muscles to force the air downward into the lower abdomen and finally into the scrotum.

Energy Exchange Exercise

In this exercise, especially for couples, the woman learns to consciously recycle potent life-force energy back to the man.

Lois Posner, R.N., certified instructor and longtime practitioner of The Healing Tao technique:

"Harnessing my sexual energy has had a profound effect on my level of health and vitality, not to mention the amazing long-term effects on my love life. With time and practice, our lovemaking grew to be wildly ecstatic and divinely inspired. We've soared to heights together that we'd never dreamed possible! It was as if our sexual union had unlocked the doors to the universe, and we came to dance across it in loving orgasmic embrace. What is most remarkable is our continued ability to transmute the lower-grade energy within us into even higher and more intensely blissful states. What an incredible gift for any relationship to be blessed with!"

Below: The Energy Exchange is a wonderful way to connect with your partner.

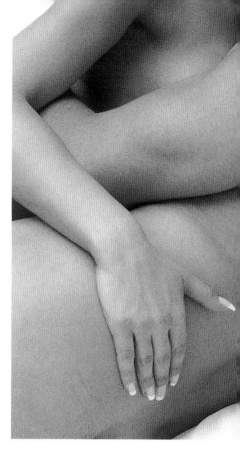

1 During the afterglow following sex, continue to lie together, with the man's tongue touching the woman's upper palate and the woman's hands resting on the lower-back (kidney area) of the man.

2 Synchronize your breathing pattern, exchanging energy flow while visually bathing your organs in the exquisite healing love that you have created together.

BENEFITS: Increases energy to the vital organs and enhances bonding between lovers.

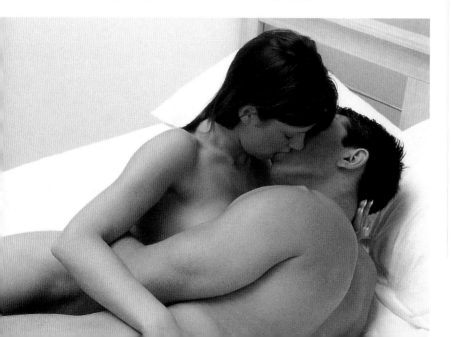

Homeopathic
Remedies

Homeopathy is a complete system of natural medicine that was brought to the Western world through the work of Dr. Samuel Hahnemann in the 1800s. Homeopathic remedies are remarkable because they seem to defy the laws of chemistry. With homeopathic remedies, the smaller the dose, the stronger the effect. In fact, chemical analysis of a homeopathic remedy will reveal that there is no measurable amount present of the substance from which the remedy was originally prepared! This thrills those people who are constantly putting down any natural protocols, even though they cannot explain away scientific studies indicating that homeopathic remedies have a profound effect.

FIND THE RIGHT REMEDY

Homeopathic remedies are a form of "energy medicine," in which a vibrational essence of a plant, gemstone, or other natural substance is instilled into a carrier substrate, such as water or saclac (tiny pellets made from milk sugar) tablets, through a process known as dilution and succussion. Homeopathic remedies are remarkably effective if the *correct* remedy is chosen. If not, the worst that can happen is that it will not work quite as well.

The homeopathic remedies mentioned below are safe to try on your own and have no known adverse effects or drug interactions. Choosing the remedy is usually done with an in-depth repertory, which describes various symptoms in great detail. For instance, if dealing with impotence, a man would consider if the condition was worse during hot or cold weather, day or night, before or after eating, and so on. There are web sites listed in the Resources section of this book that will take you through a repertory experience. Visit a professional homeopath for additional guidelines. What follows is a simplified suggestion list. You can find the following homeopathic remedies at most health food stores.

AGNUS-CASTUS: Remedies erectile dysfunction and low libido. Derived from the herb of the same name.

CALCAREA CARBONICA: Remedies premature ejaculation in men, loss of desire in women.

CANTHARIS: Increases vitality of sexual interactions. This is the homeopathic, safe version of "Spanish fly".

CARBO VEGETABILIS: Improves digestion, raises energy levels.

GELSEMIUM: Functions as a nerve-calming remedy. Its source is the jasmine, which is a romantic flower.

GRAPHITE: Helps to alleviate flatulence. Helps energize those who are debilitated.

IGNATIA: Serves as a premier remedy for grief, such as the loss of a sex partner.

LYCOPODIUM CLAVATUM: Warms up a cold, flaccid penis. Overcomes a woman's disinterest in sex.

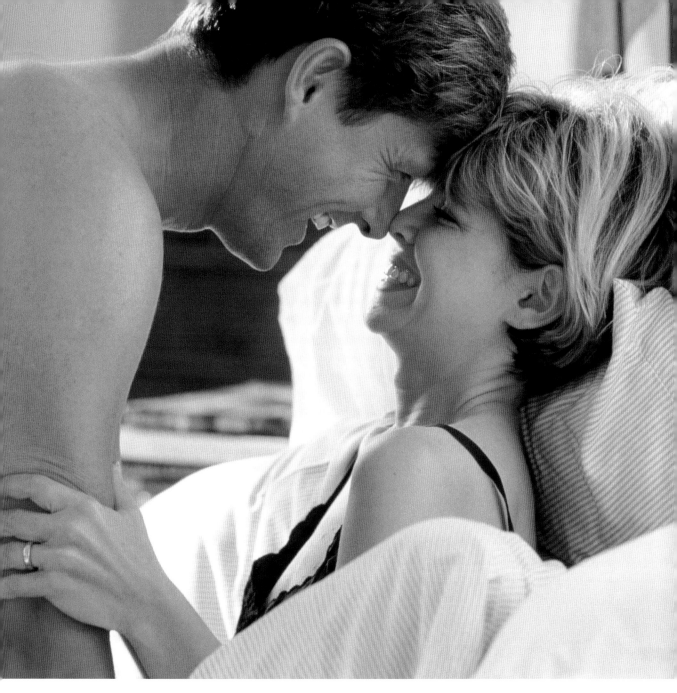

Above: Homeopathic remedies can help to alleviate sexual dysfunction in men and women.

PICRICUM ACIDUM: Overcomes sexual lethargy.

SABAL SERRULATA: Derived from the herb saw palmetto. Increases vitality of the genitals.

YOHIMBE: Derived from the herb of the same name. Increases circulation to the genitals, so that they become more effectively gorged with blood for better performance.

CAUTION

Please note that any reader taking prescription medication must be especially careful to seek professional medical attention before using any of the remedies described here.

Essence
Remedies

Essence remedies are a group of subtle energy preparations that capture the essence or energy of a plant, animal, or even an event such as a sunset, thunderstorm, wedding, or hot sexual tryst. Essence remedies can be used to increase feelings of personal power or to help open the various chakras, or energy centers, of the body.

Although there is no scientific explanation for how essence remedies work, there are many in-depth clinical reports that attest to their positive effects for thousands of people (and animals) internationally. One theory proposes that essence remedies stimulate the process of "psychoneuroimmunology"—the release of specific chemicals, called neurotransmitters, that are released in a profoundly intricate interacting network in response to every thought and action that we experience. This powerful force affects all of our bodily processes, including immune system function, cellular oxygenation, internal feelings of self-worth, and locus of control, along with the release of sex hormones.

Essence remedies are gentle and subtle. They are also totally safe and do not interact with other medicinal agents, such as prescription drugs. Essence remedies are a good choice for beginners who are starting to include natural remedies into their lives. They are also respected by advanced practitioners. Essence remedies are prepared by "capturing" the essence of naturally occurring products

and processes in water and preserving the fluid with a small amount of alcohol.

There are many companies that provide an endless array of essence remedies. I'll review a few of these, with an emphasis on the products they provide that have specific applications for sexual wellness. However, since the ability to enjoy sex is closely linked to your overall emotional state, you may want to expand your study of essence remedies to help balance all of your emotions. To use any essence remedy, place seven drops in a small glass of water and sip slowly. The remedies can also be placed directly on the skin in the same areas that perfume would be used, such as the wrists, neck, and thighs. After experimenting with prepared essence remedies, you can create your own using the techniques described below.

Bach Remedies

The Bach Remedies are the most widely available of the essence remedies, and are found in every health food store. The creator of these essences, Dr. Edmond Bach, believed that the root cause of all illness was emotional imbalance. He began to experiment with various plants that he observed to have a connection to human emotions. For instance, flowers are used to decorate weddings and funerals, while trees elicit a feeling of stability. His book

The Twelve Healers outlines the results of his research. There are now 36 Bach Remedies and many books that describe how to use them.

BACH REMEDIES FOR SEX

ELM: Lightens up feelings of being overwhelmed that relate to the responsibility associated with a sexual relationship.

WALNUT: Helps during times of transition, such as ending or starting a new relationship, or breaking ties with the past.

MIMULUS: Eases known fears related to sexual function, such as fear of pain or fear of not performing adequately.

ASPEN: Reduces vague but troubling fears and anxieties that arise for no apparent reason and may be felt in the chest and pelvis as tightness, or "armoring." Allays fears of exploring new experiences.

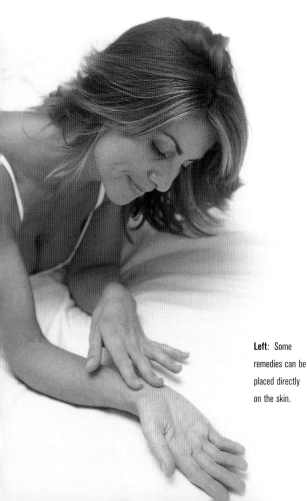

Left: Some remedies can be placed directly on the skin.

CRAB APPLE: Reduces feelings that sex is shameful. Helps promote acceptance of one's own body.

HOLLY: Helps those who are troubled by feelings of envy and jealousy because they feel they don't get enough love.

Himalayan Remedies

Drs. Atul and Rupa Shah have created the Himalayan Remedies. They are prepared from exotic flowers from the Himalayan Mountains that are infused into sacred filtered water from the Ganges River. The Shahs are Western-trained physicians who have dedicated their lives to the study of the effects of subtle energy on human health and wellness. Their remedies deal with deeper levels of psychological and spiritual imbalance, such as how to handle rejection or satisfy deep spiritual longing. Besides remedies made from flowers, they offer gemstone essence remedies and many subtle energy devices that can offset the negative effects of electromagnetic pollution and other ravages of modern life. Here are a few of their remedies that are particularly suited to creating a better sex life.

INTERPERSONAL RELATIONS AID (FORMULA NO. 23): The whole of your life revolves around interpersonal relations. This formula helps in improving harmonious relations between men and women.

INADEQUACY EASE (FORMULA NO. 41): There are times you are set back by feelings of inadequacy, when you feel negative and lose touch with your capabilities. This formula helps penetrate to the source of all capabilities and motivate the inner source of energy to accomplish the tasks of life. This formula is especially helpful for overcoming impotence and frigidity.

SEXUAL HARMONY AID (FORMULA NO. 47): This formula increases feelings of harmony, love, and desire between sexual partners.

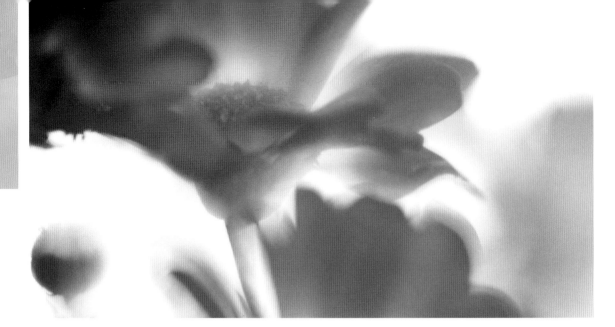

Above: Flower essences can help with emotional, sexual, and spiritual issues.

The Flower Essence Society Remedies

The Flower Essence Society, based in California, has been offering flower essence remedies for more than 20 years. The group is devoted to researching flower essence remedies and educating the public about how to use them. The society grows its flowers in biodynamic gardens or harvests them in the wild. Many of the Flower Essence Society preparations deal with interpersonal relationships, including those listed below that focus on sexual issues. These descriptions have been provided by Rainbow Resources. (See the Resources section for these groups' web site addresses.)

ALPINE LILY: Helps women who can only express their femininity spiritually to be comfortable with their physical femaleness.

BASIL: Helps to integrate sexuality and spirituality in love relationships; helps to expose the roots of sexual/spiritual and sexual/emotional conflicts in relationships and heals the stress and clandestine activities that may arise from such conflicts.

BLEEDING HEART: Addresses possessive or codependent attitudes in relationships; releases emotional attachments and heals emotional loss.

CALLA LILY: Assists with all forms of confusion about sexual identity; teaches that masculinity and femininity are balanced expressions of self within each individual.

HIBISCUS: Helps women whose sexuality has been traumatized or dehumanized to reconnect with feminine warmth and caring sexuality.

POMEGRANATE: Generates positive and balanced feminine creativity for women conflicted between career and family or men out of touch with their feminine energy.

PINK MONKEYFLOWER: Helps you to allow others to see your pain and vulnerability, and opens the heart to trust. It is especially good for those who feel a deep sense of shame, often because of childhood abuse.

QUINCE: Balances and blends masculine and feminine energies. Resolves conflicts that arise between the desires to be strong and powerful and to be nurturing and loving.

STICKY MONKEYFLOWER: Generates ability to express love in a sexual relationship. Overcomes the fear of sexual intimacy, as expressed either in repression or overactivity.

SUNFLOWER: Balances extremes of both vanity and self-effacement; heals your relationship to your father and/or masculine energies within you.

Gemstone Remedies

Essence remedies can be made from many other sources besides flowers. Gemstones are a tremendous source of energy. When quartz crystals are pressed or struck, they give off an energy field referred to as the "piezoelectric effect," which can be used to broadcast a radio frequency, run a computer, or stimulate your love life! Gemstone elixirs are either available commercially or can be prepared at home. They often address spiritual growth and matters that are connected to higher-level spiritual concerns. Gemstone elixirs can also be used to "crystallize" your sexual relationship by stimulating the glands and organs with their bright and titillating energies. Examples follow of gemstone remedies that can help improve performance.

RUBY: Brings in fiery stimulation when placed near the genitals.

AMETHYST: Increases spiritual awareness and the ability to recognize the spiritual connection with another person.

CLEAR QUARTZ: Focuses intention and clarity of purpose; increases energy.

MALACHITE: Slows you down and helps you pay attention; increases intensity of orgasms.

PREPARING A GEMSTONE REMEDY

To create your own gemstone essence remedy, select a gemstone of your choice. Soak in a glass container filled with spring water in the sunlight for a few hours. Remove the gemstone from the water with a wooden spoon. You can use this water "as is," or add a teaspoonful of brandy if you would like to save it.

Energy-Based Remedies

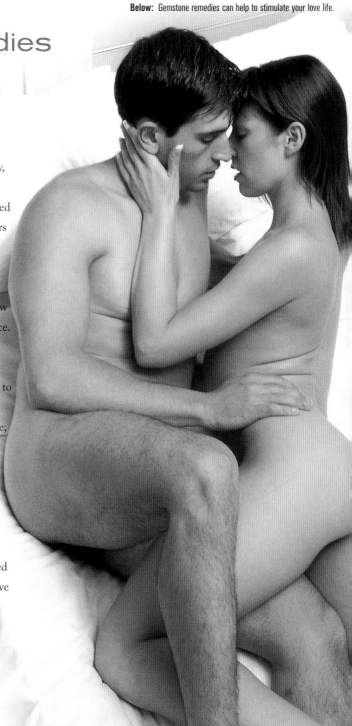

Below: Gemstone remedies can help to stimulate your love life.

Preparing Essence Remedies

After you have tried the commercially prepared essence remedies, you may want to prepare your own. The best kind of water to use is natural spring water, although filtered water will also work.

Traditional Flower Essence Preparation

To prepare a flower remedy:

1 Go outside and find a beautiful flower that inspires you. Because flowers are the sexual organs of plants, they are especially appropriate to use for creating a sexual essence remedy. Look closely at several flowers and see if there is one that actually "turns you on." Flower parts are extremely sexual and several look a lot like an open vagina or erect penis.

2 Cut the flower and let it fall into a glass vessel filled with spring water.

3 Allow the sunlight to infuse into the water for several hours.

4 Remove the plant material with a wooden spoon, or use a leaf from the plant as a spoon.

5 Add one teaspoon of brandy per pint (480 ml) of water to preserve the remedy.

6 Store in a dark amber bottle in a cool dry place.

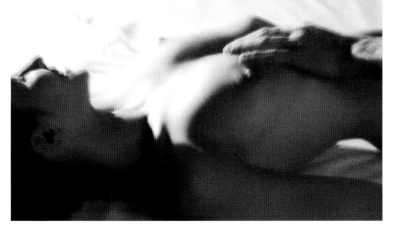

Above: Imponderable remedies can help you to save the essence of a moment.

Live Flower Remedy Preparation

Developed by Drs. Rupa and Atul Shah

This technique is different because you do not cut the flower, but rather capture its living essence while it is still alive!

1 After you identify your special flower, don't cut it off the plant. Instead, bend the flower gently into a tall glass container. Try not to crush or damage it in any way.

2 Pour spring water over the flower until it is completely immersed.

3 Allow sunlight to infuse the water for five or ten minutes, or until you "feel" the essence is captured.

4 Gently remove the flower from the glass of water without damaging it . You now have your "mother essence." Add brandy to preserve. Store in a dark amber bottle in a cool dry place.

Imponderables

Imponderable remedies capture the essence of an occurrence or a phenomenon, such as a dramatic thunderstorm, a rainbow, or the summer or winter solstice.
You can use this same method to save the essence of a special occasion, such as a wedding or a particularly erotic adventure. To prepare the essence:

1 Set a jar of water in a location in the midst of the event, such as out in the thunderstorm, on the altar during a wedding ceremony, or on the night table next to your bed.

2 Before beginning the activity, hold your hands around the jar, and project your intention to preserve the energy of the event into the water.

3 Maintain your attention for five minutes.

4 Allow the jar to stay put for several hours. Add a little brandy as a preservative, and don't forget to label the jar.

How to Use Homemade Remedies

When you purchase a prepared essence remedy, it will be accompanied by an explanation of what it can be used for. However, when you make your own, you will need to tap into your innate intelligence for instructions. Opening your inner mind to allow the influx of subtle information is a female process, whether you are a man or a woman.

1 Once you have your remedy, sit with it for a while. Have a blank piece of paper or a blank computer screen ready.

2 Hold the remedy in your hand or gaze on the flower that you prepared it from.

3 Tell yourself that your intention is to understand how this remedy can be helpful—in this case, to your sex life.

4 Breathe in and out a few times and relax completely.

5 Allow whatever thoughts come to mind to enter freely. Write them down. Don't try to force the thoughts or control them in any way. Just allow.

6 After five minutes, end the session and put the notes away. Return to them in a few hours or days. If the description feels right—it is!

CHAPTER FOUR

In this chapter, you will explore the use of the inherent life energy field as a formative force within the sexual experience. Specific techniques have been used by ancient and modern seekers, and many have found that recognizing, harboring, and directing these basic life-force energies can be effective for the conscious evolution of the individual on all levels.

Techniques for Sexual Harmony

A life-force energy pulses within and around all beings, both living and inanimate. This interconnected energy field has been described by Eastern terms such as *chi*, *qi*, and *prana*, and by Western terms such as "the bioelectric field" and "orgone energy."

Here, within these teachings, is an opportunity for growth and expansion, leading to a richer, more diverse, and more intense life experience. These teachings integrate what is thought of as "spiritual" and what is experienced as "sexual." The pulses of this energy field surround the body in the same form as a magnetic field.

When lovers join, there is an integration between their energy fields that interlaces and forms into one energy pulse being. The theory of "Open Loop Limbic Resonance" developed in the book *A General Theory of Love* describes how our brain waves and physiology are actually changed on a physical level by those we love. Changes to the immune system, hormone levels, sleep rhythms, mood stability, and other bodily functions are influenced by brain message sequencing that is emitted by other people. This is particularly true during sleep, which may explain why many people do not sleep well when their usual bed partner is away.

The orgasm has often been compared to an electrical discharge. Consider an automobile battery, which stores a large amount of electrical energy. If the two poles of the battery are connected to one another a specific "climax point" is reached and a discharge occurs, due to the flow of energy between opposite poles. Yin and yang is an Asian concept that reflects the male–female polarity that sparks a similar electrical exchange.

Yin and Yang
Energy

The Chinese concept of yin and yang describes the interaction of all of the forces in the universe. The outer circle represents the totality of existence, while the paisley-shaped, black-and-white inner halves show the interlacing interaction between the forces. The dot of the opposite color within each paisley shows that each half cannot exist without the other. There is a constant flow between the two, with each eventually becoming the other.

Yin and yang have opposite characteristics. Although many people know that yin is "female" and yang is "male," men and women both have yin and yang characteristics. Some characteristics associated with them are shown in the box below.

You can strive to bring about a balance of yin and yang energies within yourselves. Also, the strengths and weaknesses of each individual within a couple may balance the yin and yang energy between them. In some instances, the female may be stronger (yang) while the male may be submissive (yin). If there is an overall imbalance, emotional, spiritual, or physical problems can result. Too much yin, in an individual or in a couple, leads to cold, which can manifest as frigidity and impotence. If yang runs too high, it can increase anger and irritation between a couple, or lead to a fever or high blood pressure.

Below: Yang is male and yin is female.

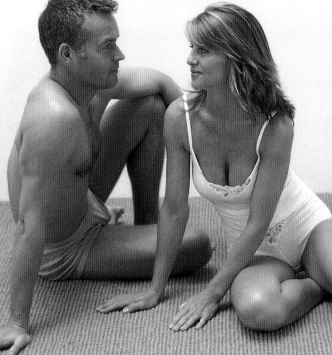

YIN	YANG
Dark	Bright
Passive	Active
Downward	Upward
Cold	Hot
Contracting	Expanding
Water	Fire

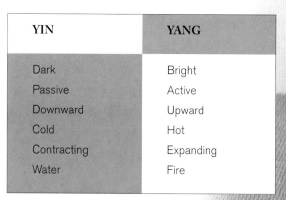

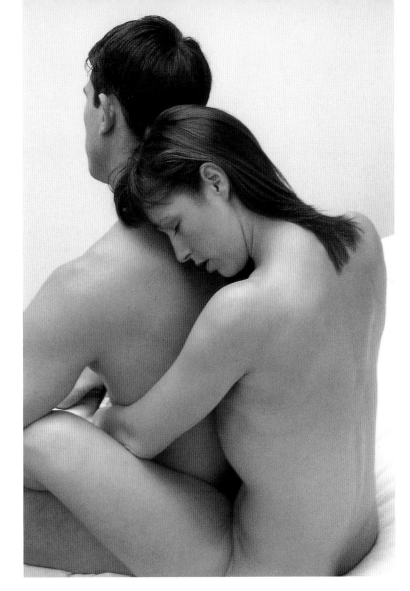

Above: All men and women have both yin and yang qualities.

pressing up against his back, her legs around his lower hips, and her body pressing against his backbone.

3 She reaches around to the front of his body and holds his penis in her hand. The exercise can continue whether or not he gets an erection.

4 Both partners begin to breathe in unison.

5 The woman strokes the man's penis, while imagining that his penis is actually attached to her body.

6 Allow the hot, strong yang energy to feel like it is emitting through "her" penis.

7 Change places, with the man sitting behind his partner.

8 Breathe in unison again, while the man holds the woman's breasts in both his hands. He can caress them with a circular motion and feel "his" breasts as if they are attached to his chest, allowing their soft, sensual yin nature to emanate through his being.

The exercise can end there, or you can choose to allow this yin and yang exchange to evolve into a full-fledged sexual session, maintaining the consciousness of being the opposite sex. As you fondle your partner's erogenous zones, imagine that you are experiencing the sensations. Couples have reported having mind-blowing orgasms following this exercise, and a closer relationship as well.

Yin and Yang Balancing Exercise

On a large piece of oaktag (a large piece of thick, shiny paper commonly used for arts and crafts projects), draw a yin–yang symbol. Take turns coloring in the paisley sections. While you are working on this, say to your partner:

"I honor the yin within you. I honor the yang within you."

As you say this, think about the aspects of this person that express yin or yang. For instance, your partner may be a male (yang) who tends to feel cold (yin), or a female (yin) who tends to be angry (yang).

1 With the yin–yang symbol in full view, the man sits on the edge of the bed with his feet on the floor.

2 The woman sits behind the man, with her pelvic bone and her breasts

Tantra

antra is a Sanskrit word that translates loosely to "weaving." This is appropriate, because one of the ultimate goals of tantric sexual practices is to weave, or interchange, souls with a sexual partner in order to experience the duality of existence within one lifetime.

Tantra refers to a large body of ancient Indian spiritual texts and to the practice and philosophy that they encompass. The tantric life includes specific practices and disciplines that weave a thread between the mundane, the spiritual, and the magical aspects of life. The female essence is highly regarded in this teaching, and both men and women participate equally on all levels of this spiritual path. Some terms that are used in tantra include:

CHAKRAS: Swirling energy power centers that surround and integrate into body systems.

NADIS: Energy channels similar to meridians in Chinese medicine.

SIDDHI: Mystical or magical power, often developed as a result of the practice of tantra.

MANTRA: Sacred sound, often repeated over and over to create a harmonious vibrational tone. "OM" is a common mantra.

YANTRA: Artwork that is viewed as a meditation device, to help visualize the sacred. The Sri Yantra combines masculine and feminine aspects to symbolize unity.

KUNDALINI: This energy is often depicted as a snake that is curled up in the sexual center. The root word *kunda* means "reservoir." The goal is to "awaken" this serpent power and allow it to rise to the higher centers, up the spinal column, into the mind's eye. This brings enlightenment.

YONI: The feminine aspect. The yoni, or "sacred place," is the female sexual organ. It is hidden, internal, mysterious, soft, receptive, and embracing. When it pulses during orgasm, it is the source of universal life-force energy.

LINGAM: This is the Sanskrit name of the male sexual organ. The translation means "Wand of Light." The lingam is revered and honored in the tantric system and is considered a sacred channel of pleasure and life-force energy.

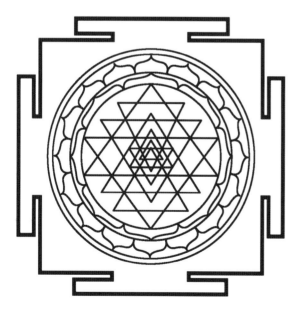

Above: The Sri Yantra. The upward triangles represent the Shiva (female) principle, the downward, the Shakti (male) principle.

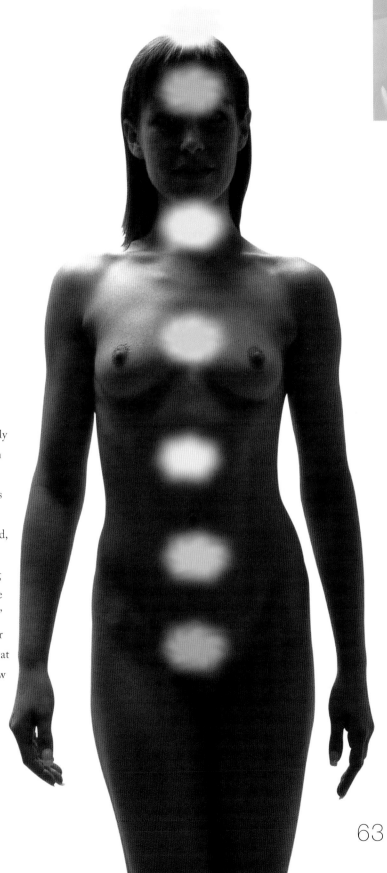

Tantra teaches various methods of learning to use breathing techniques, mantras (sounds), and visualizations to awaken the kundalini. Some practices are done alone and, once mastered, practiced with an adept partner.

KUNDALINI ENERGY

Occasionally, the kundalini energy may be released by a couple during lovemaking, even though they have not been consciously attempting to do so. This may be felt as an earthmoving, breathtaking experience. There are reports of people feeling anxious and overwhelmed if they release the kundalini before they are properly prepared, but generally it is a positive experience.

In many ancient teachings, including tantra, the breath is considered the essence of life. Meditations to generate "inner fire" and other tantric techniques use the power of the breath. On page 64 is an exercise that you can do with a lover to increase the flow of mutual orgasmic energy.

Right: The seven chakras of the body. Each chakra is an energy center that surrounds and integrates into the body's systems.

Techniques for Sexual Harmony

Sexual Bifocus Breathing

In many ancient teachings the breath is considered the essence of life. Myths in several ancient traditions speak of a powerful being breathing life into inanimate objects. Breathing techniques are especially important in yoga exercises and in Buddhist and Hindu meditation practices.

Meditations to generate "inner fire" and other tantric techniques use the power of the breath. Some breathing patterns are believed to help specific organs and systems in the body, such as aiding digestion and stimulating the sexual centers. Here is an exercise that you can do with a lover to increase the flow of mutual orgasmic energy.

Below: Sit back-to-back with your partner for step 4.

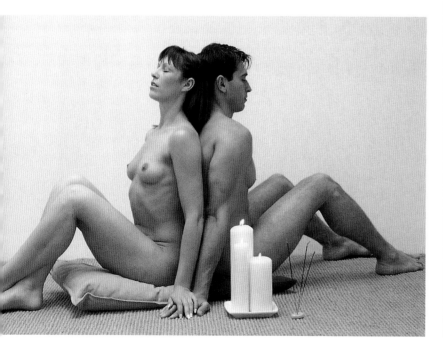

Gather the following in a comfortable quiet space:
Large pillows
White candles
Incense
2–5 quartz crystals (at least 1–2 inches/2.5–5 cm long)
Sexual lubricant (massage oil or similar)

1 Choose a comfortable room, preferably with a rug or carpet on the floor. Each person should sit on a large and supportive pillow.

2 Light some candles. White is the preferred color, since it emphasizes air energy.

3 Light some incense. Champa incense is perfect, because it intensifies the energy flow out of the body. However, feel free to make other choices of colors and scents.

4 When the room is prepared, sit back-to-back with your partner. Line up the bases of your spines, so that the hollows in your lower backs (and your base chakras) are touching.

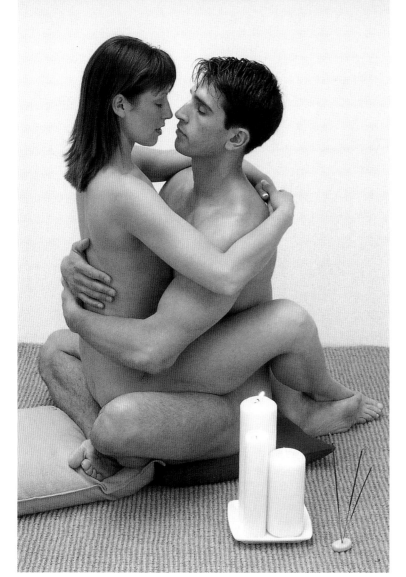

Left: Sit intertwined, chest to chest (step 10).

onto each other's genitals, while you continue to breathe in a synchronized rhythm.

10 Arrange yourselves in an intertwined position. One partner sitting on the other's lap works well. If the male's penis is erect, it can be inserted into his partner's vagina.

11 With legs intertwined, press your chests together, allowing the heart chakras to touch.

12 Place a quartz crystal between you at the point where your chests are pressed together. You can each hold a quartz crystal in one or both hands as well. Crystals will intensify the exchange of energy and increase your perception of the experience.

13 Wrap your arms around each other. Visualize a golden light energy coursing between you.

14 As you squeeze the crystals in your hands and between your heart chakras, a piezoelectric effect—a spark of electrical energy—is created. Direct this energy with your inner vision until you both feel totally energized. After five to eight minutes, release the crystals. You can continue into a spontaneous lovemaking session that is likely to end with a super-energized mutual orgasm.

5 As you breathe in, visualize your breath coming in through your nose, traveling down your spine, exiting through your base chakra, and entering into the base chakra of your partner. As you do this, your partner should do the same. Continue this breathing exercise for three to five minutes, or until you both are experiencing a warm or tingling sensation in the lower spine.

6 When you are both experiencing this sensation, signal each other by touching hands.

7 Focus your breathing in the middle of the back, in the area of the heart chakra. Press your backs together at this point and continue to send the energy of the breath out of your heart chakra and into your partner's heart chakra, while your partner does the same.

8 Continue until you both experience warmth or tingling in this area.

9 Turn around so that you and your partner are facing each other. Gently massage the sexual lubricant

Kabbalah

Kabbalah is an ancient Hebrew teaching that enables practitioners to act in accordance with universal principles, leading to a harmonious and balanced life. Kabbalah recognizes the interconnectedness of all aspects of reality: physical, emotional, and spiritual. It strives to bring these forces into balance by "walking the middle path." One of the symbols of kabbalah is the tree of life, which symbolizes the polarity of all things in the universe, including male and female.

Understanding and practicing the concepts of kabbalah reinforce the idea that sexual desire is a wellspring of creative energy that emanates from the soul's desire to connect with another being in a mystical integration of life forces. This conscious and aware connection is far superior to mechanical movements performed by people who are disconnected from the higher spiritual splendor of sexual intimacy. Kabbalah teaches that the lover's embrace is like an electrical spark that transcends the mundane world.

In *Sacred Secrets, The Sanctity of Sex in Jewish Law and Lore*, Rabbi Gerhson Winkler explores the celebratory attitude toward sex that is ingrained in ancient Jewish literature. According to kabbalistic teaching the libido, or sexual drive, is a powerful formative force that can be used as a positive motivational current. Rabbi Winkler shares the age-old attitudes toward human sexuality that he claims have been distorted in modern times.

The teachings of the kabbalah explore sex as a source of pleasure rather than being only a condition for procreation. Kabbalistic texts, such as *The Zohar*, share specific teachings on both the sanctity and the joy of sexual relations, and specifically encourage sex as a celebration, such as during the holy sabbath and on other festivals and holidays. Kabbalists believe that there is a spiritual connection with the divine during sacred times and that this connection can be tapped into through the divine connections between two lovers, if sex is peformed with a conscious spiritual intention.

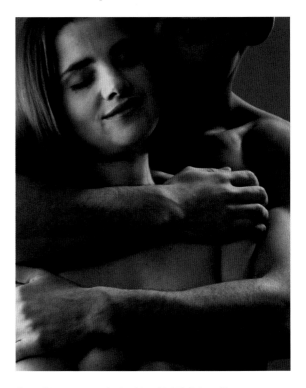

Above: Enjoying your sexuality is celebrated in kabbalistic teaching.

Chapter Four

Orgone
Energy

Orgone energy is the name that physician/researcher Wilhelm Reich, M.D., (1897–1957) used to describe the life-force energy as expressed as sexual energy.

Reich further developed the concept of orgone energy. While a student of Sigmund Freud, Reich became familiar with the concept of libidinal energy, which Freud described as a "psychic" field. Reich expanded on this idea and discovered that this energy was not only experienced on a psychological level, but could actually be measured and documented with scientific instruments, such as the oscillograph.

Dr. Reich measured the bioelectric sexual charge that develops between two sexual partners. He quantified this energy and discovered many fascinating aspects of the phenomenon of sexual sharing. Reich found that the electrical charge that emanates from the body increases when an erogenous zone is stimulated, but only when the stimulation is experienced as pleasurable. If the same individual perceives the same stimulation technique as unpleasant or annoying, there is a corresponding decrease in the oscillograph reading. A person can accurately predict if the reading would increase or decrease, as a direct result of the degree to which he or she felt pleasure, or, conversely, the lack thereof. The presence of an obvious outward sign of sexual arousal, such as an erect penis, would not automatically indicate an increase in the

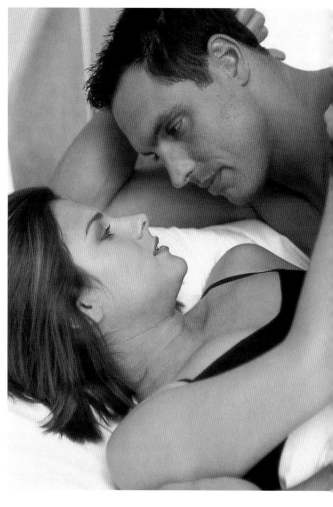

Above: According to Reich, lovers produce a measurable bioelectric charge.

bioelectric reading, unless it was accompanied by a pleasurable experience.

Reich theorized that the lack of ability to fully experience sex as pleasurable was often caused by "armoring." Armoring is the development of tight, blocked areas within the physical body, often in the muscles, which is caused by internalizing negative emotional experiences. If a person has unresolved issues— especially if linked to negative sexual feelings that developed during childhood or other times—there exists a corresponding block in the musculature. Reich also believed that as orgone energy builds up in the body, it must be released regularly, or it could lead to tension,

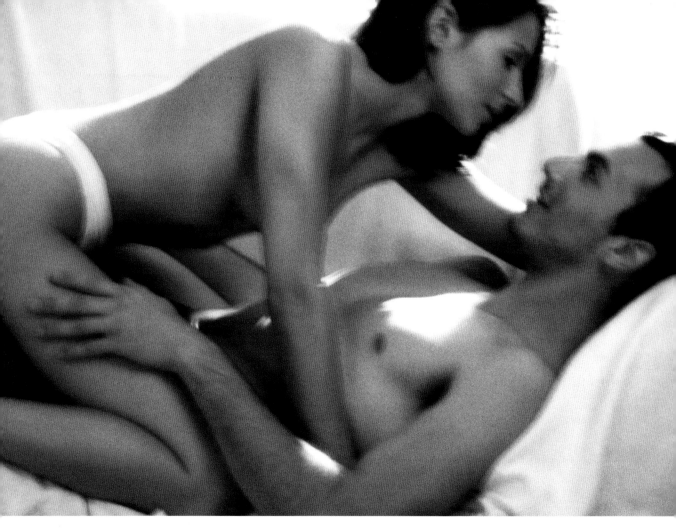

Above: Orgone energy needs regular release through pleasurable sexual intimacy.

nervousness, irritability, and other psychological and physical symptoms. He believed that unrepressed pleasurable sexual release was necessary for health and that regular orgone accumulation was important for revitalizing the system and increasing strength and longevity.

ORGASM—A BIOELECTRIC CHARGE

Reich considered the orgasm as a bioelectric phenomenon that was similar to the charge and discharge of a battery, although in order for a full discharge to occur, sex had to be experienced as pleasurable. He envisioned both the male and female circulation as the source of the bioelectrical charge, the penis as an electrode, the female lubrication as an electrolyte-conducting solution, and the vagina as another electrode. In Reich's words:

"The male and female circulations and the mutually stimulating plasmatic excitations in the autonomic nervous systems represent the inherent sources of electrical charge on the organs of sexual contact. The equalization of the potential gradient occurs between the two surface potentials—penile epidermis and vaginal mucosa."[1]

Two important terms that describe orgone energy are "or" and "dor." They represent two different sides of the same energy force:

OR: (ORGONE) is the positive, life-enhancing aspect of ORGONE energy.

DOR: (dead ORGONE) is the negative, life-depleting aspect of ORGONE energy.

Too much orgone energy can become dor, and decrease overall health, vitality, and sexual stamina.

Chapter Four

Make Your Own Orgone Accumulator

Orgone energy can be harvested and used to increase your energetic biofield. Here are instructions on how to put together a homemade orgone accumulator, such as an orgone box and an orgone blanket. Commercially available orgone accumulators and orgone generators can be found on-line (see the Web Resources section).

ORGONE BOX

Cardboard box (any size)
Gold spray paint

Use any cardboard box. Spray paint the entire box, inside and out, with gold spray paint. Cover the box with seven layers of paint, allowing each coat to dry for 24 hours before applying the next coat. The orgone box can be used to "charge" objects that you intend to use in specific ways. Place meditation objects, such as feathers and crystals, inside the box for later use, or experiment with a few dildos and other sex toys to bring an added "charge" to your love nest.

ORGONE BLANKET

Make an orgone blanket by creating layers of organic and metallic materials. Have four pieces of high-quality pure wool material cut in 4 x 4 pieces. For added energy, use wool that has been dyed specific colors that attract sexual energy, such as red or orange. Have three sheets of steel wool prepared. The round steel wool pads that are sold for use on commercial floor cleaners work well; they can be spread out into a square shape. Now layer the wool and steel wool together, with the wool as the top and the bottom layer, for a total of seven layers. Sew the edge together all the way around.

Many people say that they can "feel" the orgone energy if they sit on the blanket for five to ten minutes. The experience may be felt as a slight tingling sensation, or as a gentle warm or cool breeze.

Use the orgone accumulator sparingly. Do not use for more than half an hour at a time, and not more than one hour total per day.

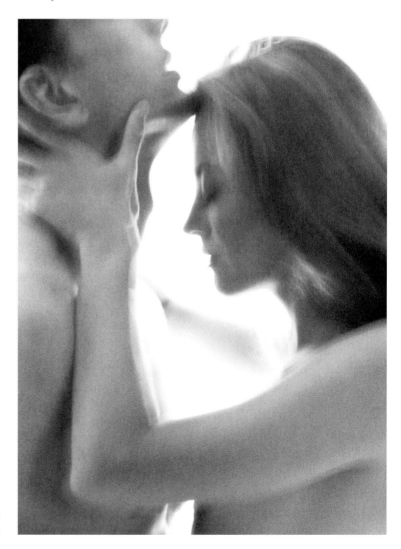

Right: Orgone energy may be experienced as a tingling sensation.

5

CHAPTER FIVE

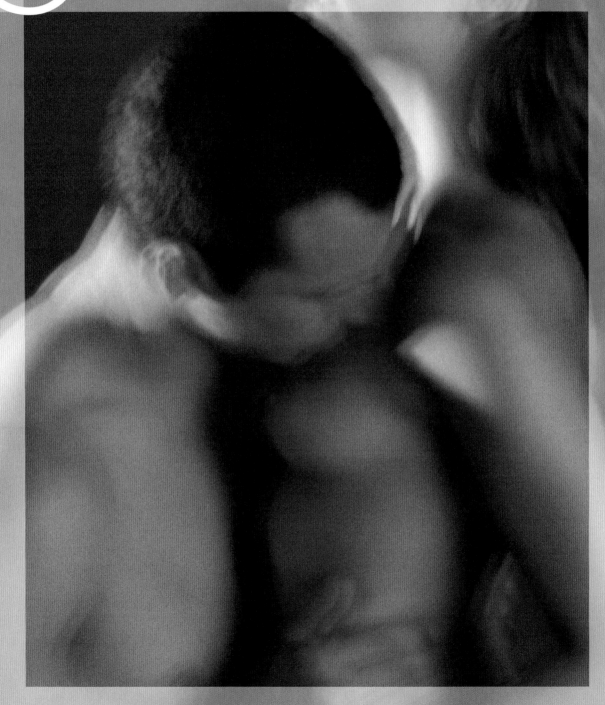

In the pages that follow, you will be shown how to awaken your senses of sight, sound, touch, and smell, so that you can increase awareness and heighten all aspects of your pleasure centers.

Titillating the Sexual Senses

The fact that we have five senses may be a coincidence; or could it be part of a divine plan? After all, five constantly appears in nature: we have five fingers and toes; Eastern culture refers to the five elements—air, wood, metal, fire, and water; Feng Shui, the Chinese art of placement, centers around five colors, five directions, five animals, and five types of energy; the occult has the five-sided pentagram as a central figure. In fact, five appears in all major religions and philosophies as a number of sacred importance.

We explored taste in Chapter 2. Here, we will look at the other four senses and explore a variety of ways to become more aware of the rich complexity available through each sense. By expanding the sensitivity available through each of the senses, you can elevate the sexual experience to new heights as you integrate your expanded perception and understanding. In addition, these exercises help to heighten the sense of pleasure you can experience by bringing your mind and body into harmonious balance.

You can explore your relationship with color as you take the color test and understand the science behind viewing erotic visual stimulation (as well as enjoying it!). Visualization and fantasy can be very strong sexual tools. One psychiatrist interviewed more than 4,000 people, and found that men under 25 have sex on their mind at least once every two minutes, and women of the same age, once every five minutes. Thus our "inner eye" is certainly involved with sex on a regular basis!

Murmur in your lover's ear and know how important the sensuality of your voice is, while you listen to the rhythm and harmony of the energy between you.

Learn how to give and receive a sensual massage and investigate the ancient touch therapy of acupressure and the "footsy" technique of reflexology.

An incredibly evocative sense, smell is very important in sexual attraction. Indulge in the rich aromatic sensuality of aromatherapy essential oils while you share elevation of all of your senses.

Sight

Astonishingly, two-thirds of all the information that is contained in your brain comes from input to the eyes. The eyes capture light energy that is then interpreted by the brain as a vision. Indeed, the age-old saying, "beauty is in the eye of the beholder," holds especially true for sexual attraction.

Color

Color has a profound effect on our emotions and moods. Much has been written about the use of color when "dressing for success" or planning a particular kind of environment. For instance, research indicates that painting the inside of jail cells pink helps to calm inmates who are held for a short time, but increases aggression in those who are kept in the cell for a longer period. An area of a city where prostitution is common has been called either the "red light" or the "blue light" district. Our own sexual profiles may also be determined by our color preferences.

Below: People drawn to the color black may have extreme sexual preferences.

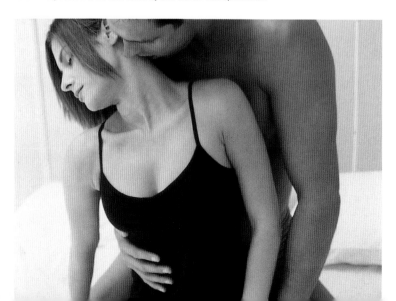

Color test

The following is an exercise you can try alone or with your lover to see how your own color preference fits your sexual personality.

INSTRUCTIONS FOR USING THE COLOR CHART:

Look at the colors below. Immediately choose your three favorite colors, without taking any time to decide—just go with your first spontaneous response. Then turn to page 74 to read the description of the type of sexual partner you make.

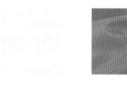

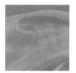

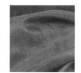

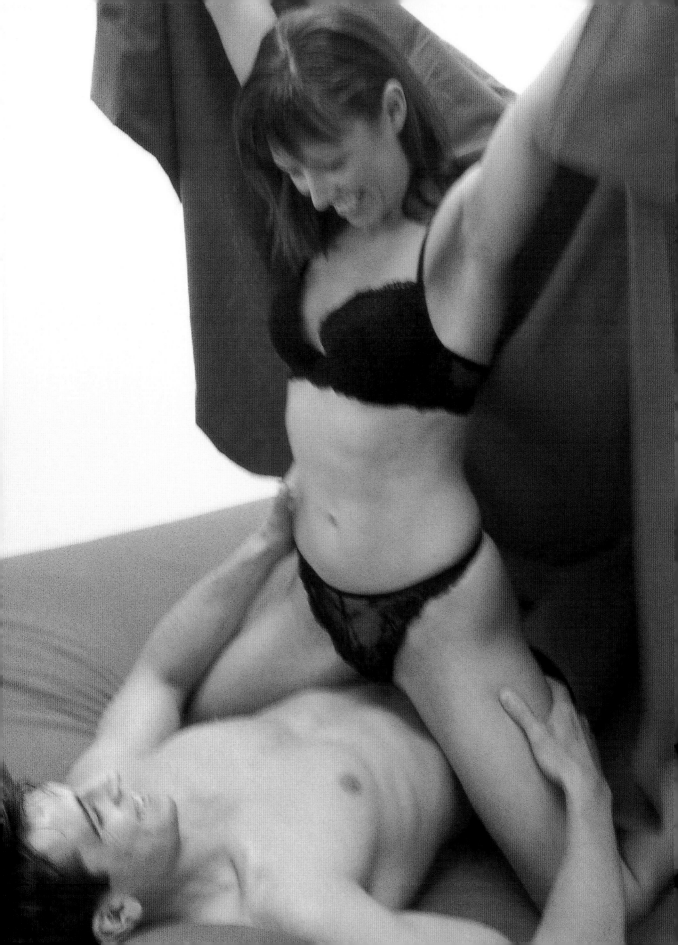

WHITE If you are attracted to white you may have an issue with sex being pure. White is a puritanical color and you may think that sex is appropriate only within a heterosexual marriage and for procreative purposes.

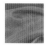

RED People who are drawn toward red tend to be hot in their sexual preferences. This includes walking on the wild side and being uninhibited in bed. They often enjoy pure lust, which does not have to be associated with love, and may not be into commitment to one partner, of either the same or opposite sex. They may also enjoy group encounters and other exotic erotica.

ORANGE If orange is your color choice, you tend to be a romantic, interested in lavish, long foreplay. Setting the stage is all-important and an orgasm is only the icing on the cake. You may be unrealistic in your approach to long-term love, becoming disenchanted when the orange glow fades after the initial first few encounters.

YELLOW People who choose yellow will have a more intellectual outlook on sex. You will not usually choose a bed partner simply because of strong emotions, but will evaluate the situation from a "mind's-eye" view. This may inhibit your arousal and pleasure, but plays out well for long-term commitments.

GREEN Those who choose green are coming from a balanced perspective. Green is in the middle of the color spectrum. It is a supportive color, and lovers who choose this color are grounded and loving, although probably not dazzling in their performance. The "green" lover can be depended upon as a loyal "one lover" partner.

BLUE If you choose blue as one of your favorite colors, your love partner is in luck. Blues are nurturing lovers, combining the best attributes of highly developed techniques, designed to satisfy their partner, with the openness to enjoy a full, passionate orgasmic experience themselves. At the same time, they can love deeply, and can be wonderful lifetime partners.

PINK Pink people, both men and women, have a childlike exuberance for sexual delight. They often like to remain "players" well into advanced age, enjoying multiple partners, and light, noncommitted relationships. They enjoy the flirtations and fun that accompany initial meetings, but pass on the seriousness and depth that are needed to sustain anything long term.

PURPLE If you are attracted to purple or violet, you are more involved with the spiritual than the physical. Sex may seem like a carnal occupation that is beneath you, unless it is engaged in for the purpose of spiritual revelation. You may want to include certain rules and standards to sexual encounters to meet your goals, which often focus on your own orgasm, rather than having a sexy good time.

BROWN Brown is the ultimate earth tone. If you chose brown, you are a reliable and steady lover. Browns focus their attention on their lover's needs, and are hopeless romantics. A night home by a cozy fire, sharing massages, and creating a slow burn, which will end in a satisfying climax, is preferred to a noisy nightclub and a quick "flash in the pan."

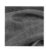

BLACK People attracted to black may like their sex outside the usual boundaries, enjoying extreme sexual practices. If this is not your style, shy away from those who choose black.

Visual Stimulation

Sexual artwork has been a cultural norm for most human civilizations around the world. Both the tiniest miniature erotic sculptures from China and huge monolithic Hindu temples in India are frequently decorated with an endless variety of sexual interactions.

Scientific evidence proves that viewing sexual images is arousing. The stimulation occurs in a particular part of the brain (the right prefrontal cortex) and messages are then sent to the genitals. Brain scans show significantly increased activity on men after they watch a sexual video than after watching a neutral one. This corresponds to an increase in the rigidity of their erections.[1]

To enjoy visual sexual stimulation as a couple, both parties must be comfortable with the experience. It is fine if the enthusiasm level is not the same. For instance, one partner may be totally excited and filled with anticipation, while the other is mildly or even shyly curious. If either party is against it, on moral, religious, or spiritual grounds, then viewing sexual images together is not for you.

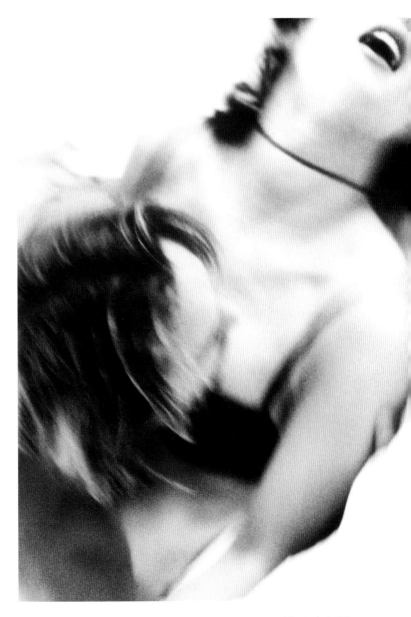

Above: Some people are driven wild by visual stimulation.

Erotic Visual Stimulation Exercise

Pick a time when you know you will not be disturbed. Let the kids stay at their grandparents' house. Take the phone off the hook and turn off the cell phone. Put your sexiest satin sheets on the bed, or throw them over the couch—wherever you will be having your private party. Then follow these steps:

1 Light incense or spray the room with aromatherapy oils.

2 Turn down the lights—use candles or red light bulbs instead.

3 Put on your sexiest clothes.

4 Have lubricants and sex toys handy.

5 Just relax, and begin to view whatever source of erotic images you have chosen.

6 Allow the images to come gently into your consciousness without judgment or expectations.

7 Take some time just to watch the "action."

Begin participating only when you feel ready. Mirroring the sexual activity you are viewing is often enjoyable and may continue or evolve into other activities as you and your partner desire.

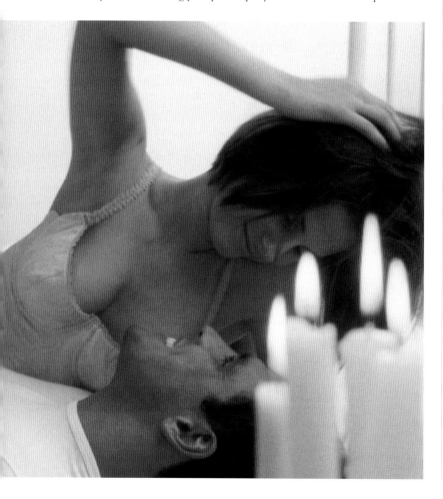

Left: Set the scene for your sexual adventure with candles and incense.

Visualization and Fantasy: "Seeing" with the Mind

Visualization is the use of the inner eye to create a movie that you can actually see, albeit with your imagination. Science has proven what ancient healers have known for centuries—that activating visualization techniques creates measurable changes in living organisms. For example, both wound healing[2] and immune function[3] are aided by mind–body techniques such as affirmation, creative visualization, relaxation, and conscious breathing, in which you focus your attention on your breath, breathing deeply and relaxing.

Sexual excitement is also greatly enhanced by the use of fantasy. Almost everyone has imagined a sexual scenario. Some people can actually reach orgasm by becoming deeply involved in the inner vision of a fantasy. When this happens during a dream (most prevalent during adolescence), it is called a "wet dream." Fantasy can be used to stimulate blood flow to activate an erection, enhance vaginal lubrication, and increase desire. Some philosophies teach that absorption in mental fantasy displaces love energy away from your "real" lover. Sex therapists, however, often use fantasy as a technique to improve sexual function. Indulging in fantasy occasionally is normal and healthy. Spiritual teachings, such as tantra, instruct the dominant lover to visualize male or yang energies, such as a volcano or fire, while the submissive partner visualizes yin or female energies, such as a valley or water. Male and female or same-sex partners can switch off on yin and yang visualizations to benefit from both roles.

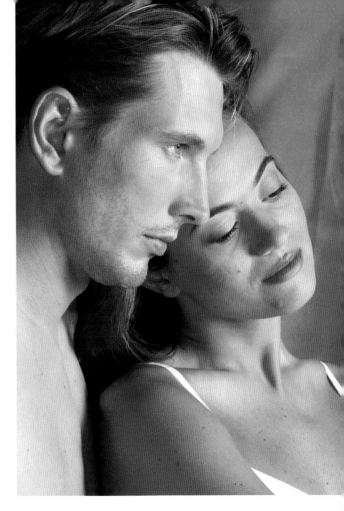

Above: Make sure you and your partner are comfortable with each other's fantasies.

Fantasies may be used before getting deeply involved in a sex session, during the heat of the action, or just before climax. Some people choose to discuss their fantasies with their partners, while others keep these visions as secret internal treasures. Both systems seem to work well depending on the person and the situation. Mind's eye fantasies are a safe-sex way to experience deep desires, and don't have to be acted out in real life in order to be enjoyable.

There are several fantasies that rate as favorites. These include homosexual encounters, making love with someone else's mate, having sex with a famous personality, being forced to have sex, and group sharing. Fantasy sex may be a problem if it has to be engaged in every time you have sex, however, rather than as an occasional diversion.

Sound

The sound of a lover's voice can be one of the most intimate sources of attraction. The voice can actually vibrate the eardrums of another person like a loving embrace. The auditory sense is as important to a positive sexual experience as touch, sight, sound, or smell. Sound can be used creatively to set the mood, seduce, and satisfy. Many people love to hear the sounds made by their lover during sex, and also enjoy their own vocalizations.

After lovers are familiar with each other, a great element of surprise can be inserted into the action by the use of sexually explicit talk. Surveys consistently show that even the most conservative people are often greatly aroused by their lovers saying "naughty" things in bed. This technique can serve as a safe release for sharing sexual fantasies as well as a direct method for turning up the heat.

If you are too shy to openly express what you would like to say, try reading a passage out loud from a sexually explicit book that mirrors what you have in mind. That way, you can gauge your partner's response while enhancing your own comfort level.

Phone sex is a wonderfully erotic foreplay technique and great to use if you are far from home, but also useful to work up to a hot time that very evening. Find a quiet area to call from. Tell your lover exactly what you are going to do to him or her when you get him or her in bed. Be very specific, and be ready to carry it out the next time you are together!

Once you are actually involved in a sex session, the best way to approach the use of verbal eroticism is to be sure the language matches both your own and your partner's comfort level. The use of strong sexual slang might be extremely stimulating, or it might be a complete turnoff; ask ahead of time, or just try it and gauge the reaction.

Although there are those "silent types," most people vocalize loudly during sex, unless they have to keep it down due to kids or neighbors. It can start as a low gasp or crooning hum, and escalate into loud vocalizations like screams, grunts, or shouts—sometimes accompanied by curses or prayers!

Purposely mimicking animal noises is often a turn-on. Pretend you are both cats or lions, and purr or roar accordingly. The ancients believed that a baby's spirit would be imbued with the characteristics of a particular animal if the parents mimicked the animal's movements and sounds during sex. The same may be said for your relationship. Do you want the strength of a lion, or the sweetness of a dove? Practicing animal sounds will bring out the true animal nature in both of you.

The Mysticism of Vocalizations

Ancient Chinese, tantric, and Taoist texts all recognized the importance of the sounds of lovemaking. The yoga text *Ananda Raga*, a sex manual written in 1172 C.E., describes the use of specific sounds that can help raise the

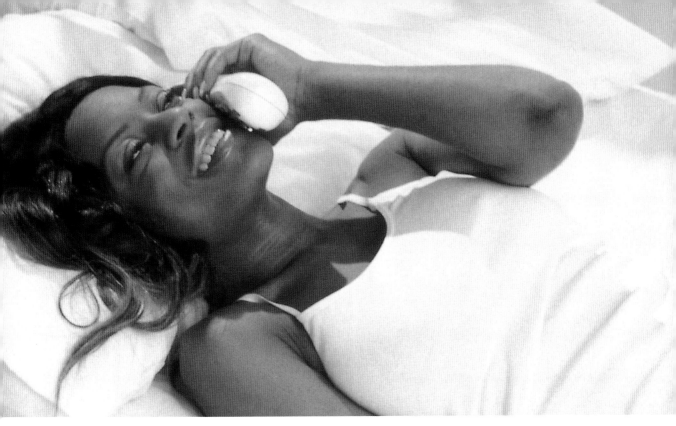

Above: Phone sex is a great way to get into the mood.

level of the sexual experience to connect with spiritual ecstasy. Here is one you can try.

The sound "eh-vong" is a mantra that can be used to balance the duality of energies between the male and female. While engaged in a sex session, incorporate the use of this mantra instead of just vocalizing ad lib. Use the breath, and let the sound ride on the inhalation and exhalation. You can use this mantra out loud, or just focus on it in your mind.

A wonderful time to use mantras is during the afterglow cool-down period. You can breathe in and out with your partner and say the mantra together.

Music's Role in Cultivating Sexual Energy

This section contains contributions by Steve Angel, D.C. (see page 124).

Music has profound effects on our physical, emotional, mental, and spiritual well-being. Almost everyone has experienced the effect of music on mood. Music relaxes as well as inspires and is able to stimulate an extraordinary range of emotions, from blissful pleasure to extreme sorrow and despair. Music has directly measurable physical effects; it can raise or lower blood pressure and heart rate.[4] Perhaps most important, music can profoundly alter our state of consciousness. This realization has been used by shamans and healers from all indigenous cultures. The extremely diverse power of music can move us from tears to joy, from pain to pleasure, and even from disease to healing.

There is much current research that indicates music can affect our immune function response[5] and function as a stress reducer. Music can heal, inspire, stimulate, and even seduce. Most interesting is music's relationship with sexual activity and sexual selection.

Music as an Aphrodisiac throughout History

"... it appears probable that the progenitors of man, both male and female, before acquiring language, endeavored to charm each other with musical notes and rhythm."
Charles Darwin[6]

Throughout history, music has been recognized as a potent aphrodisiac. Humans communicated with music before language existed. Music created in the form of simple rhythms and melodies was used to attract the opposite sex during mating and sexual selection. Darwin asserted that human music arose through mate choice:

> "All these facts with respect to music and impassioned speech become intelligible to a certain extent, if we may assume that musical tones and rhythms were used by our half-human ancestors, during the season of courtship."[7]

Drumming and other rhythmic beats have traditionally been used as part of fertility ceremonies in different cultures throughout the ages. History reveals that music holds a special place of vital importance for sexual matters during the Ancient Greek civilization. Aphrodite, the Greek goddess of sexual love, was said to have been attracted to beautiful and alluring music.

Modern Music and Sexuality

Rock and roll is one modern genre of music where an obvious sexual overtone can be seen between the performers and the audience. Groupies follow their favorite bands on tour and fight each other to procure sexual adventures with the musicians. Jimi Hendrix was alleged to have had sexual liaisons with hundreds of groupies, while maintaining parallel long-term relationships with at least two women and fathering at least three children in the United States, Germany, and Sweden, before his death in 1970 at the age of 27. Elvis Presley swiveled his hips in an obviously sexual gesture, causing women to literally swoon and, at times, lose control and attempt to physically attack him. Hip-hop stars typically grab their genitals while romping across the stage.

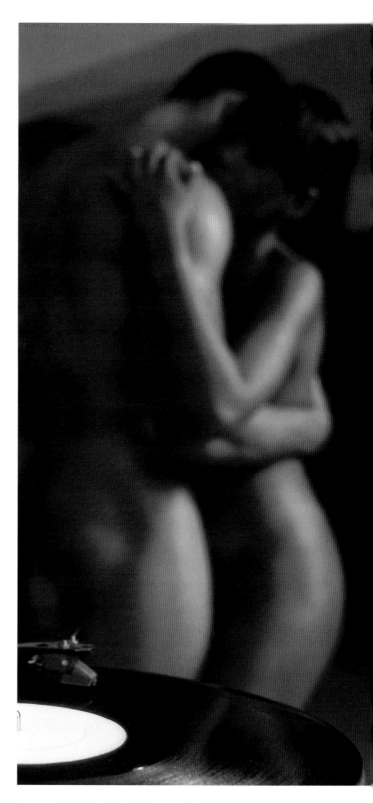

Above: Many couples enjoy making love to their favorite music.

However, rock and other forms of music with loud and rapid drumbeats may not be the best listening choices during a sexual encounter. Although it may act as a sexual stimulus initially, the overall effect can impede a lovemaking session. Instead, music that has a gradual, slow increase in tempo, such as Ravel's *Bolero* and many blues pieces, can be more effective in building up sexual energy to a slow burn that ends in an ultimate orgasmic crescendo.

Rhythm and Harmony

The term rhythm describes the number of cycles or beats that occur in a given amount of time. The motion of the tides, planets, and stars, as well as the pulse of the heartbeat, are all governed by the law of rhythm. In music, rhythm is determined by the beat. Harmony occurs when there is a smooth synchronicity between the various pulses within any rhythm. Rhythm and harmony are the elements of music that are stimulating sexually. The beat of a piece of music can induce dance and movement even without the use of sexually provocative lyrics. Lovemaking can be described as a form of dance that culminates in the final gesture of orgasmic release and then relaxes into the warm afterglow. The rhythmic harmony between lovers can determine if the experience feels smooth, comfortable, and satiating.

Each of us has a unique and natural rhythm. When we are in harmony, life seems smooth and simple. Different people have different rhythms, as expressed by the phrase "she dances to the beat of a different drum." Part of the sexual attraction between partners is the often "chemistry," an allusive quality that can often not be explained. We may describe a particular skin color, hair color, height, and other physical factors that we usually find attractive. However a person with that exact description may leave us cold while someone else who looks quite different may be very attractive to us. Part of this mysterious attraction mechanism is tied into the natural rhythm of our prospective partner and how it interacts with our own to create harmony.

Many couples find that making love to music enhances the experience. Others find that the sound of music interferes with their own natural rhythm and harmony, which can change during a particular lovemaking session. Some people report that they enjoy having music on at first, but like to keep the remote handy and turn it off once things get steamed up.

Try different types of musical accompaniment, both alone and with a partner, to determine the effect on you. The most intimate of all communication can occur during sexual sharing, which allows for organic communication to occur on multiple energetic levels of being. Adding the use of sound to your sexual repertory can add to the intensity and fulfillment of your love relationship.

Erotic vocalization

Here is an exercise that can help bring both partners into a seething state of excitement:

1 Tell your lover exactly what you intend to do next, before you do it. Say, "Now I am going to run my hand down your inner thigh." You can vary this by saying what you are doing, while you are doing it: "I love to watch you get excited while I touch you here." Adding a blindfold worn by the recipient turns this exercise up a notch.

2 Ask your partner to tell you exactly what he or she would like you to do. This is exciting to both parties, and can help you learn what brings your lover pleasure. Communicating specifics can be done outside of the love nest as well, but some people will share more about their true desires during the vulnerable state of lovemaking.

3 You can also use the voice as a love instrument. Humming into the scrotum or along the shaft of the penis, or on top of the mons of a woman, will bring gasps of pleasure. (Those gasps are also part of the use of voice sounds during sex.)

Touch

Touch is the sense that is most intimately and obviously involved in sexuality. The one thing most people long for, when they find someone sexually attractive, is to touch them. The skin, which is the body's largest organ, is covered with sensors, tiny nerve endings that are always "on." They enable you to experience pain, heat, and cold as well as pleasure.

The most marvelous feeling that exists can be the feeling of a lover's touch, whether that involves a slight brushing of the skin with the fingertips or a full body embrace during lovemaking. That wonderful total exhalation—releasing tension and becoming filled with peace and pleasure—occurs when we sink into our lover's embrace. According to the famous Victorian author and philosopher, Thomas Carlyle:

> *"There is an important temple in the universe and this is the human body. Nothing is more complex and more saintly than this divine form. We reach, without knowing, the heaven and the divine happiness when we touch with our hands the lover's body."*

Many aspects of touch can be used consciously to enhance a sexual experience. Sharing a massage is a wonderful, sensual experience that both relaxes and sensitizes all of the body's nerve endings. It can be used as a kind of extended foreplay, slowly building into a very hot sexual experience. The ancient arts of acupressure and reflexology are fantastic tools to explore. They can increase your ability to stimulate erogenous zones and have a healing effect at the same time. All areas of the body can be used as "touching tools." Experiment with using just your elbow, knee, or earlobe to explore every inch of your lover's body.

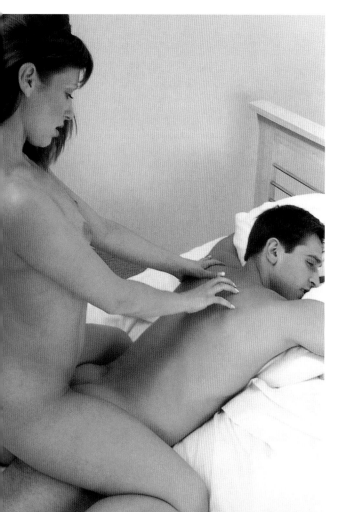

Left: Touching your lover can be a wonderful, shared sensuous experience.

Chapter Five

Finger Length Sex Hormone Evaluation Technique

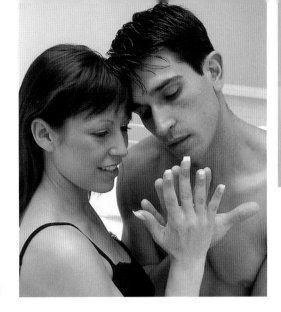

Above: Men and women's hormones are revealed in their finger lengths.

Of course, the hands are the body part most often used for touching and the hands themselves may hold a sexual secret. Amazingly enough, just looking at your own and your lover's hands can reveal a clue about your sexual selves, as explained in the exercise that follows.

This amazing phenomenon is not ancient folklore, but has been scientifically investigated. Research has shown that the same bit of the genetic material, DNA, provides information to the body about the formation of the hands at the ends of your arms as well as the genitals at the end of your trunk. After finding out about this genetic blueprint, researchers of the Population Biology Group at the School of Biological Science, University of Liverpool, decided to see if there was a measurable connection between finger length and sex hormone levels. Dr. Manning's team studied 400 males and 400 females ranging in age from 2 to 25. The results indicated that women, on average, have longer index fingers, while men tend to have longer ring fingers, which also correlates to sex hormone levels (see right).

The wedding ring has traditionally been placed on the fourth finger in civilizations as old as ancient Egypt.

The hands have also been recognized in other cultures as holding "secrets to the soul." Palmistry is the art of reading the lines on the palm of the hands, which can give you and your lover a lot of information about your sexual relationship. Using a book on palmistry, hold your sweetheart's hand and run your fingers down his or her love line to check your compatibility. You may be fascinated by what you learn.

While you are paying attention to your hands, you may want the added advantage of learning to perceive and influence your own and your lover's energy field, by practicing the Hand Energizer exercise on page 84.

1 Hold up your right hand.

2 Compare the length of your index finger (the one next to the thumb) and your ring finger (the fourth finger, the one next to the pinky).

MAN
Right-hand ring finger longer than index finger:
• Higher testosterone
• Higher sperm count

WOMAN
Right-hand ring finger shorter than index finger:
• Higher estrogen
• Higher levels of other female hormones

Hand Energizer Exercise

The palms of the hands can be energized and used to project a strong energy field to yourself and your lover. You can learn to consciously extend (or contract) this energy field. Here is an exercise that can make your energy field palpable so that you can more easily learn to work with it. This exercise may be done alone or with a partner.

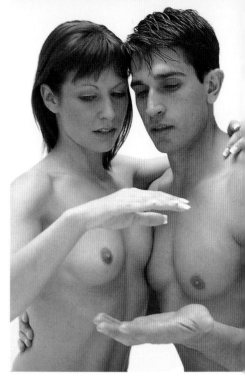

Above: Experience the energy of your lover's hands.

1 Sit alone, or across from your partner, on a straight-back chair.

2 Place both feet solidly on the floor, hip-width apart.

3 Be sure all distractions are at a minimum. Turn off the phone!

4 Start to breathe deeply, allowing your lower abdomen to totally relax and completely fill with air.

5 Feel your breath extend down through your lower abdomen and then down to where your seat meets the chair.

6 Extend the breath down through your thighs, your legs, and through your feet into the ground.

7 Once you are taking slow full breaths, rub your palms together and rotate them in a circular motion seven times, while you feel your breath flowing into your palms.

8 Separate your palms, and then bring them very slowly back toward each other, but do not allow them to touch.

9 Continue breathing while you allow yourself to "feel something" in between your palms. People describe this feeling as tingling, heat, or pressure, as if a ball is between your palms.

10 Pull your palms away from each other once again, and then bring them back toward each other. Often the distance between your hands will be farther apart than before, at the point you begin to feel the "energy ball" between them.

11 If you have a partner, interlace your palms with each other without actually allowing them to touch. Slide your hands in and out and around each other, while you both continue to breathe. Your hands will now be energized.

For an erotic variation, perform this exercise nude or with only minimal clothing. After building the energy fields, run your hands over erotically sensitive areas of the body, stimulating them without touching, by extending the energy tendrils through your hands and fingers over your lover's body.

Finger Foreplay

The fingertips are infiltrated with a myriad of nerve endings, and are an extremely sensitive extension of our erotically attuned anatomy. Kirlian photography is capable of taking a photographic image of the energy field that extends from the fingertips.

You can focus on your lover's fingers to enjoy a secret sexual exchange while you are in a public place, such as the movies or at a party.

You can play "gender benders" while performing this activity, by imagining yourself being either male or female and then switching roles in your mind. This can help to balance yin and yang energy.

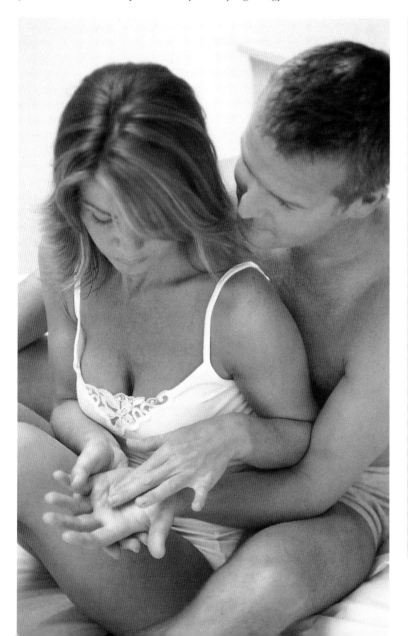

1 Hold your lover's hand gently in yours.

2 Begin to massage each finger and gently stroke each finger up and down.

3 Imagine, while you are doing this, that the fingers are actually the genitals. Imagine each finger to be a small erection.

4 Encircle each finger with a ring formed by the thumb and first finger, and slip this ring around your partner's finger, gently inserting the finger and then sliding it in and out.

5 Occasionally circle the tip of one of your fingers around in a circle on your partner's palm.

Left: Touching and massaging your partner's hand can be a very intimate experience.

Sensual Massage

The most important thing to know about massage is that everyone can do it. Although it is best to see a highly trained, licensed massage therapist for medical or therapeutic massage, all lovers can learn enough about the basics to give their partner the benefit of relaxation and stimulation that a sensual massage can bring to lovemaking. A massage can be a be-all and end-all in itself—for instance when one partner is not up to having sex, but still would like to share on a physical level. Or, it can be an enticing extended foreplay, moving from the most gentle stroking to the most intimate and erotic probing.

Have a quiet time and place set aside. Clean towels and all-natural massage oil are important. Choose an oil from the health food store that contains only all-

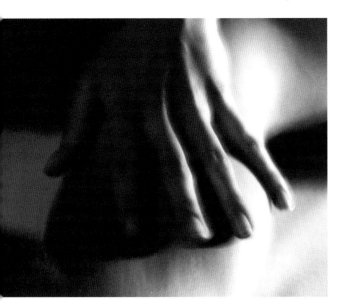

natural ingredients, or make your own by combining organic sesame oil and any of the delicious essential oils that are discussed in the Scent section (see pages 90–95), such as lavender or rose. You can also sprinkle a few drops of an essence remedy into the massage oil to enhance the emotional healing (see the Essence Remedies section in Chapter 3). Warm the oil to body temperature, especially in cool weather. The last thing you want to do during massage is "shock" your lover's skin.

You can start with your partner on his or her front or back. Allow him or her to breathe deeply and relax, while the "giver" does the same. It is always best for the recipient to be covered by a sheet to maintain warmth. Body temperature tends to go down while receiving a massage. You can disrobe the part you are working on, and then cover it when you are finished. Strokes can vary from long and light to deep and circular. The more you practice, the more you will become comfortable with various strokes.

You can begin with the head and face. This area holds a lot of emotional tension, especially around the temples. Continue down the throat and upper back and shoulders, depending on whether you are starting with the recipient placed up or down. As you continue, be sure to do everything bilaterally; spend an equal amount of time on each arm and leg. Don't put too much pressure on the bones of the spinal column. Work along the sides of the vertebrae. The area of the lower back, where the kidneys are located, is especially important. Many people

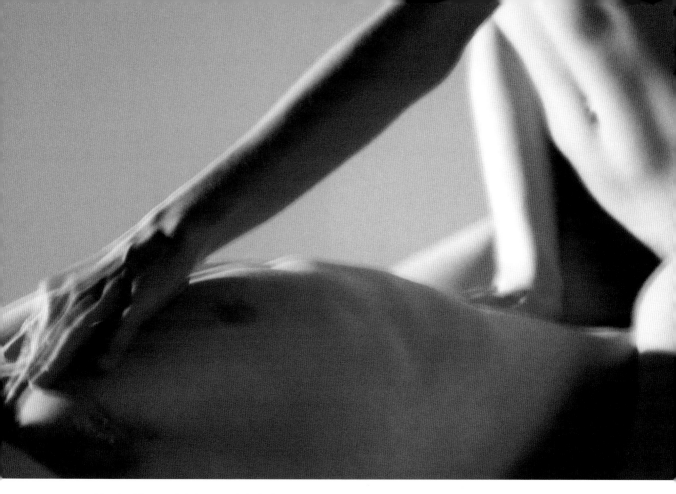

are sensitive in this area. It is intimately linked to sex because, as traditional Chinese medicine recognizes, kidney energy is linked to sexual energy. Knead the kidney area gently, and energize the area by rubbing your hands together until they are warm. Then place the hands firmly on the kidney area, hold them there, and begin gently rocking your partner's body side to side. This is a very nurturing move.

If you find massage fascinating, there are videos and classes where you can learn more specific techniques. Meanwhile, do what feels right. Exchanging massages is one of the best ways to learn what your lover enjoys. When you are the recipient, pay attention to what feels especially good to you, and then use that same stroke on your partner, when it is your turn to give.

Communicating verbally during a massage is important. The recipient can help by allowing the giver to hear a subtle groan of pleasure or a quiet, "That's a little too much pressure," which can help to refine technique.

Above: Sensual masssage can be just that–a massage–or it can be foreplay.

When doing a sensual massage, you can practice the Hand Energizer exercise described earlier in this chapter to further enhance the massage by adding energy balancing to the physical comforts of massage.

After you are both feeling relaxed, the massage may move toward a more erotic adventure. This does not have to happen. A massage exchange can be an ultimately fulfilling and complete experience in and of itself. However, between lovers, a sensual massage can be a wonderful prelude to the most dynamic erotic expression. Allow the hands to explore erogenous zones, very lightly at first, and then with increasing pressure. Gauge your partner's response, or ask him or her what he or she would like you to do. Let your imagination run wild. The combination of scented oil, trusted sharing, relaxation, and nerve-ending stimulation started by the massage will surely end in a passionate scenario.

Acupressure

Acupressure is an ancient system of Oriental healing that is based on stimulating meridians—energy channels that run throughout the body in specific patterns connecting various areas of the body. Acupuncture points are specific points along these meridians that can be used to unblock energy, diagnose specific illnesses, such as appendicitis,[8] and help with impotence.[9]

Blockages along the energy pathways interfere with the function of internal organs that are connected to that particular meridian. Acupressure is the system of helping to unblock the meridians by massaging acupuncture points along the meridian, which helps to stimulate circulation of body fluids, such as lymph and blood, as well as the more elusive energy that flows along the meridian. Acupressure is a worthwhile study to help balance all areas of health, but in this section we will discuss a few of the acupressure areas that are particularly effective in enhancing sexual wellness.

THE SPLEEN MERIDIAN The spleen meridian begins in the big toe, then runs up through the groin and on to the chest, passing right near the nipple. Stimulating this meridian by gently rubbing along its length, focusing a little extra pressure on several of the acupuncture points as you go, increases the flow of energy to the sex organs.

THE SEX CIRCULATION (PERICARDIUM) MERIDIAN To stimulate the sex circulation meridian, massage your lover starting at the armpit, down the forearm, along the

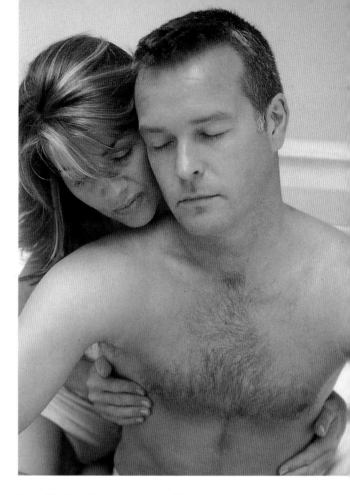

Above: Stimulating points along the spleen meridian increases energy to the sexual organs.

inside of the wrist and palm, ending at the tip of the middle finger. Gently suck the finger at the end of this move to entice and excite!

THREE-MILE POINT (ST 36) This point is located on the leg along the stomach meridian. Stimulate it on both legs simultaneously. It helps to restore "yang consciousness," which alleviates fatigue and increases sexual desire.

SHENSHU POINT (BL 23) Stimulate this point on both sides of the lower back. It nourishes "kidney yin." This is an important concept in traditional Chinese medicine, which links the strength of the kidneys with sexual energy.

FRONT MU POINT—ZONGJI (CV 3) Located where several of the meridians come together, this point fortifies kidney energy and greatly benefits sexual health.

Reflexology

Reflexology is an ancient art that evolved in cultures all over the world. It is fascinating to discover reflexology charts in ancient Egyptian hieroglyphs, cave drawings in Spain, and silkscreens from China, all of which depict a similar theme.

During a reflexology treatment, pressure is applied to areas of the hands, feet, and earlobes—the "thinnest" parts of the body—in order to positively influence internal organs. Pressure on these external areas is believed to relieve blockages that inhibit energy flow and circulation to the internal organs. By allowing a free flow of energy and circulation, the organs are rejuvenated and balanced. In addition to the areas already mentioned, the penis can be massaged as a reflexology organ. Although there is no hardcore scientific proof that massaging reflexology points helps heal internal areas, the massage itself is relaxing and reduces stress. The following reflexology charts highlight a few of the areas that are most closely associated with sex.

Front
Mu
Point

Pericardium

Three
Mile Point

The
Spleen
Meridian

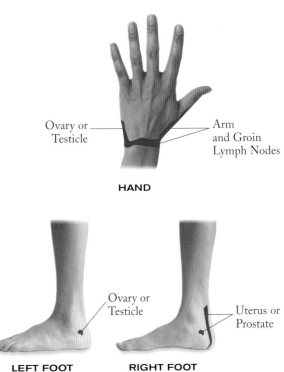

Ovary or
Testicle

Arm
and Groin
Lymph Nodes

HAND

Ovary or
Testicle

Uterus or
Prostate

LEFT FOOT

RIGHT FOOT

Scent

The sense of olfaction—the stimulation of nerve endings in the nose—is more closely linked to emotional reactions than any other sense. Entering a room with the pleasant aroma of cooking can bring tears of joy to the eyes of most people if their childhood home had a similar aroma when their mother or grandmother was preparing a special meal. The part of the brain that regulates the sense of smell is located within the limbic system, which also houses the seats of emotion and sexuality.

What is considered a good or a bad smell is influenced by cultural norms. For example, in medieval times men going off on journeys pleaded with their women to abstain from bathing until their return, so they could look forward to a strong welcome-home aroma. Sigmund Freud postulated that modern Western culture's obsession with hiding natural body odors was part of the armoring process that leads to dysfunctional psychological states. Interestingly, one study found that while married men preferred a minty, clean breath smell, college men found an odor of alcohol on the breath most enticing.

Most living creatures—plants, insects, and animals alike—use the power of scent to initiate and insure successful sexual encounters. Flowers release scented oils that are often specifically designed to mimic the sexual scent of a species of insect, thereby enticing a visit by the insect, accompanied by the very pollen that flowers need in order to reproduce.

Pheromones are a class of chemical produced specifically to act as sexual attractants. The word pheromone comes from a Greek root word that means "excitement carrier." Until recently, the common belief was that humans had evolved beyond communicating through the sense of smell. However, science has now uncovered evidence that humans produce, release, and react to pheromones.[10] Pheromones cannot be perceived as a scent by most people. In a sense, they are "secret" messages that influence our behavior without our conscious awareness.

THE IMPORTANCE OF PHEROMONES

Men release pheromones such as androstenol and exaltolide, although the amount varies from person to person. The vaginal fluid of women contains pheromones called copulins. It seems that woman are more influenced by both perceptible odors and the more subtle pheromones than men. For instance, women tend to be up to 1,000 times more sensitive than men to the aroma of musk. In clinical trials, men who applied an odorless lotion containing commercially prepared male pheromones found that women were more affectionate and more willing to join them in sexual encounters. Whether this was due to the pheromones or due to an increased sense of self-confidence in the men, has not been resolved, however.

The vomeronasal (VNO) organ, also called Jacobson's organ, exists in most species of mammals and

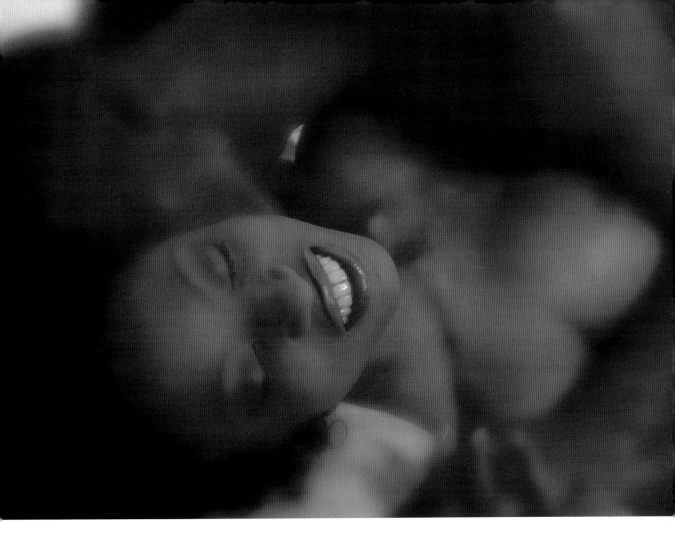

Above: Pheromones can drive lovers wild!

is known to play an active role in creating social order as well as influencing sexual behavior. In humans the VNO is located at the base of the nasal cavity. It has been known to exist in the human fetus since the Dutch surgeon Roysch described it 1703, but scientists believed that it was vestigial (no longer used) and inactive in adults. However, the human VNO is now believed to be an active organ that is sensitive to pheromone stimulation. In the insect and animal kingdoms, an exotic array of complex activities are known to stimulate the VNO. For example, more than a hundred species of insects and the largest mammal, the elephant, have a pheromone chemical in common, called (Z)-7-dodecen-1-yl acetate, which elicits a sexual response among members of a given species.

When animals interact, they will usually sniff the sex organs of the animal they encounter. This stimulates the Jacobson's organ. Current theory supports a similar, if more subtle, system of humans "checking each other out" through the VNO.

FOOD CHEMICALS AND SEXUAL ATTRACTION

A tantalizing discovery has been made that shows that several foods that have been used for their aphrodisiac powers for many centuries, such as truffles and oysters, contain chemicals similar to human pheromones. According to the Smell and Taste Foundation in Chicago, the smell of pumpkin pie and buttered popcorn are sexually stimulating to men, and the aroma of licorice turns women on. Other scent stimulants include doughnuts for men and baby powder and, not surprisingly, chocolate for women.

Titillating the Sexual Senses

Essential Oils and Aromatherapy

Essential oils have been used by humans since ancient times for stimulating the olfactory center. Essential oils have healing properties beyond the aromatic stimulation that they provide. True aromatherapy oils are lipophilic or "fat-loving" substances that can be transported across the skin and into the bloodstream. Therefore, deliciously scented aromatherapy oils can be used many ways, both to stimulate the olfactory organs, and increase sexual drive and pleasure. Only true essential oils—pure distillations that do not include any kind of man-made chemicals or preservatives—can be used in this manner. When choosing essential oils, use pure oils from a health food store or order them from a high-quality aromatherapy manufacturer. Commercial products that contain chemicals and fillers are often labeled as "Aromatherapy" but they are not the right choice. Read the label carefully, especially the "other ingredients." Pure essential oils have no other ingredients.

There are many ways that essential oils can be used to set the mood and increase sexual pleasure. Of course, you have to sniff them to choose your favorite.

- Sprinkle a few drops of oil on a light bulb before turning on the light. The heat from the bulb will fill the room with a delightful aroma.
- Create an aromatic spritzer: Fill a 2-ounce (56 g) spritzer bottle with spring water, add five drops of an oil of your choice, or a combination of several. Spray around the room, and on yourself and your lover.
- Add five to ten drops of any combination of oils to a warm bath, along with one-half cup of baking soda and one-half cup of sea salt.
- For direct massage, add a few drops of essential oil to a base oil, such as sesame or almond oil. Essential oils are too strong to put directly on the skin, especially delicate mucous membranes.

Below is a listing of several essential oils that have proven to be sex helpers. Experiment with each oil that you feel attracted to. Then add several together to create your own special blend.

CLARY SAGE

This has a nutty, sweet fragrance. The name is derived from the Greek root word *claris*, meaning "clear." It was used as a healing oil during the Middle Ages. Germans added it to wine to improve the flavor and the English brewed it into beer. Its aphrodisiac properties may be due to its ability to relax muscles, which can reduce menstrual cramps, backaches, and help combat insomnia. It is calming and sedating.

JASMINE

Jasmine has a sweet, rich, exotic floral aroma. It is often available as an "absolute," extracted with alcohol, rather than a pure oil. Derived from the Persian *yasmin*, this flower was used by many cultures (including Indian, Arabian, and Oriental) as a scent for religious as well as

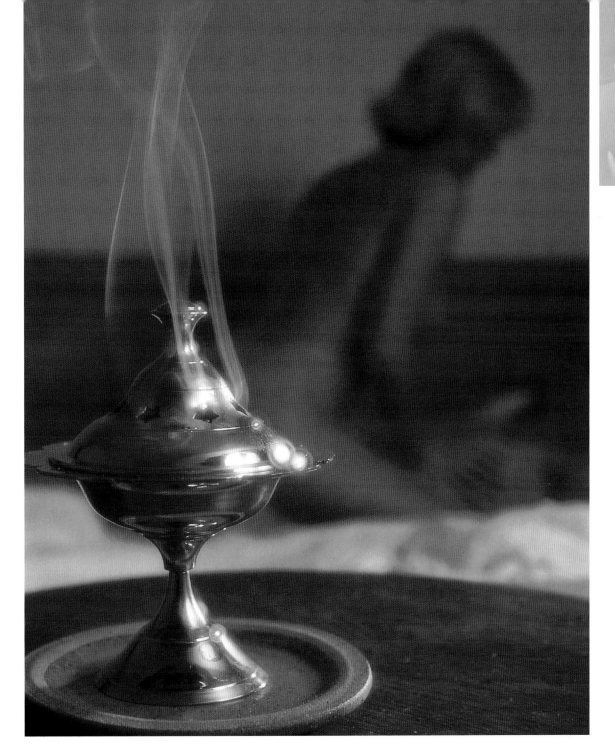

sexual rituals. Legend claims that jasmine opens the heart chakra and brings favorable forces together in a love relationship. It can help to soothe frayed nerves and improve the mood, as well as restore energy. Sexual issues such as frigidity, impotence, and premature ejaculation can be aided by this calming flower.

LAVENDER

Lavender has a fresh, light, clean aroma and is one of the most popular aromatherapy oils. It has been rated repeatedly as the number one aphrodisiac scent. *Lavera* means "to wash" in Latin, since it was a favorite as a bath oil for the Romans. The flowers were thrown on the floor, and released antimicrobial oils when walked on. It was believed to solidify feelings of desire between partners and to ensure fidelity. Lavender is said to increase blood flow to the sex organs, increasing the power of a man's erection as well as clitoral sensitivity in women.

MUSK

This essential oil has a scent that is manufactured from an animal extract rather than a flower. It is produced by the male deer of the *moschus moschiferus* species, which lives in the Himalayas. These small deer have two sacs under their bellies that produce the "musk balls" during mating season. In ancient times, only kings and other royal gentry were permitted to use musk, which was often rubbed

Below: Rose petals have a long association with love and attraction.

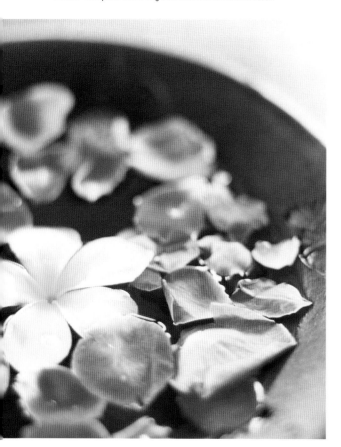

directly on the hair or beard, to impart to the wearer extreme personal power, both sexual and social. The Koran mentions the use of musk for sealing the "drinks of paradise." Musk was combined with honey and ground rubies in Ayurveda, the traditional medicine of India, to bring vitality and energy to the user. Today, the scent is used as a sexual attractant that is added to perfumes and colognes. Try combining musk with sandalwood and patchouli for an exotic erotic atmosphere.

NEROLI

Neroli is also called "orange blossom" and has a floral, sweet scent. Neroli is pricey because it takes approximately 1,000 pounds (454 kg) of orange blossom to make one pound of neroli oil. Anne-Marie de Tremoille, the Countess of Nerola, was rumored to have preferred this oil to perfume her bath; hence, the name. Brides traditionally have worn orange blossoms in their hair, and the scent is intimately connected to the marriage bed. Neroli is also good for the skin and soothes and relaxes.

ORANGE

Orange has a tangy, sweet, fresh smell and is helpful for stimulating the entire system and adding energy to any intimate encounter. It opens up emotions and allows for unrepressed sharing, as well as forgiveness. It is said to bring happiness into marriage, and to act as a de-stressing scent.

PATCHOULI

Patchouli has a sensually rich scent that is spicy and musty-sweet at the same time. It has a direct association to lust and mysterious eroticism. In Malaysia and India, the name patchouli comes from the Hindustan words for "green" and "leaf." It was used as an insect deterrent in goods shipped from the Middle East to England. Patchouli is a wonderful scent for older lovers because the scent of patchouli itself improves with age, like fine wine. It has antiaging properties such as healthy skin rejuvenation, and acts as an antioxidant, as well as reducing stress and anxiety.

Chapter Five

ROSE

Rose exudes a scent that is full and flowery. The name *rose* may be derived from the Greek *roden*, which means "red." Rose has been recognized as an aphrodisiac since earliest human times, and Aphrodite, the Goddess of Love, favored this flower. Rose is universally recognized for its intense romantic value, is a favorite for showing loving intention, and also has a connection to the spiritual— rosary beads were made from rose petals! Flower girls often scatter rose petals down the aisle at weddings as a symbol of love, attraction, and sensuality. True rose essential oil is quite costly because it takes 180 lbs (81 kg)—60,000 roses—to extract an ounce of rose oil. In addition to its sexually stimulating properties, rose oil can ease female menstrual irregularities.

SANDALWOOD

Sandalwood has a distinctive scent that is rich, earthy, and exotic. It conjures erotic visions of *The Arabian Nights* and belly dancers. Sandalwood was used more than 4,000 years ago by members of desert caravans who traveled from India to Rome, Egypt, and Greece. The teaching of tantric yoga recommends this scent for awakening the sexual energy of the kundalini (see the section "Tantra" in Chapter 4). In addition to its widespread use as an aphrodisiac, especially in cases of impotence and frigidity, sandalwood has antiseptic and calming qualities.

TUBEROSE

Possessing a heavier scent than rose, tuberose is quite a different plant. It has white flowers that resemble the lily. Tuberose is used as an aphrodisiac less for its romantic properties than its ability to enhance pure lust. It is marketed as a cut flower used for decoration as well as a source of essential oils. It can help balance the reproductive system in both men and women.

VETIVER OIL

Vetiver is dark, with a fresh, spicy scent. The grass of this plant has been used as thatch housing materials in tropical

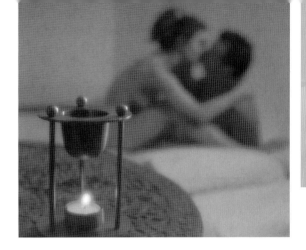

Above: The tangy scent of orange is said to bring happiness into marriage.

areas, and it freshens the room air as well as discouraging insect invasions. Perhaps this is why it is credited with evoking a sense of security in relationships and is called the "oil of tranquility." It has both calming and stimulating properties, perfect for relaxing and having energy for a sexual adventure.

YARROW FLOWER OIL

With its spicy, sweet aroma and light color, yarrow was used as a charm against evil spirits in Scotland. It helps to improve circulation. A compress of diluted yarrow flower oil can be pressed on hemorrhoids for astringent action to help shrink them and bring relief. This same compress can be applied to the penis when flaccid to improve circulation for more powerful erections. It can also help menstrual disorders. Yarrow is said to solidify love relationships by raising self-confidence and opening the heart.

YLANG YLANG OIL

Ylang ylang has a sweet, deep exotic aroma. The name *ylang ylang* means "flower of flowers," and it was used in Europe to prepare macassar oil for the hair, to impart shine and encourage illustrious growth. The flower petals have traditionally been used in Indonesia to cover the wedding bed, thus imparting good luck and lust for the honeymooners. Ylang ylang's aphrodisiac properties stem from its antidepressant and relaxing effects, helping to put people "in the mood."

CHAPTER SIX

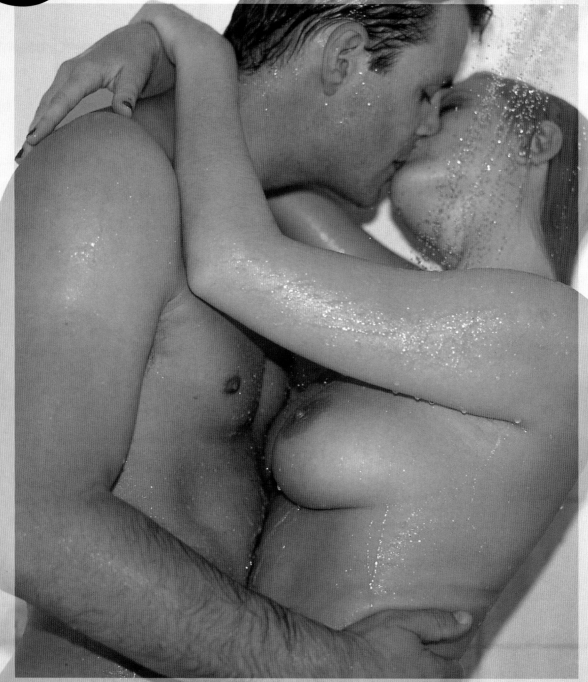

In this chapter, we look at some of the many love magic recipes and rituals that have been successfully used by men and women for thousands of years. Many of them involve the use of body fluids, such as menstrual blood and semen. Others combine herbs with gemstones, metal mirrors, water, and earth. Some of these activities are done by one person alone, often to bring them the object of their desire. Others are performed as a couple and are meant to build up the attraction between the two people involved. The session may or may not end in a sexual union.

Rituals For Sexual Magic

When you work with magic, you produce a standing energy wave that you send out to the universe to make your intentions manifest into physical existence. By performing magic rituals, you focus the energies of your total being by planning, gathering necessary tools, creating a sacred space, and investing your time and attention. This awakens your inner being to the importance of the outcome of this activity. The real magic is the intense power of the mind.

Magic is a general term that can have many different meanings. In a general sense, magic is an attempt to interact with and influence energy fields through the use of focused consciousness, ritual, and prayer. In this chapter, you will explore the use of energy interventions that are considered "love magic."

Prepare yourself physically and spiritually before beginning to put together any ritual or recipe. Choose special articles of clothing that you wear only during the times you are doing this special work. Bathe before beginning, using your powers of visualization to cleanse both internally and externally, so that you enter the sacred session with a clear mind and a clean heart. Use a special scented soap, such as lavender or patchouli, which you use only before doing rituals.

Working with magic ritual is a very powerful activity; you will truly reap what you sow. It is a good idea to have a special altar set up in your home where you can keep your sacred symbols, such as stones, jewelry, photos, or any other objects that you collect over time and that "speak" to you. This ritual preparation will put you into a "twilight" state that increases your receptivity to cosmic energies outside the realm of ordinary reality. It connects you to the archetypal consciousness of mystics and shamans, and activates the use of your will.

Being in sync with the astrological aspect of the planets can strengthen the power of your magic. The planet that most strongly relates to sexual attraction is Venus, especially if romance and love are involved. Mars is also involved with sexual energy, especially pure lust. Friday is the day of the week most receptive to couple energy, and is the best time to work sex magic, although you do not need to feel restricted to this time schedule.

Aloe Vera Ritual

to Attract a New Lover or Strengthen a Couple's Bonds

The following ritual involves the herb aloe vera. Aloe vera has a very slippery inner gel that is similar to sexual fluids, particularly natural vaginal secretions. In fact, aloe vera gel can be used directly on the genitals as a sexual lubricant. Aloe vera was considered to be a religious symbol in Egypt, and both Muslims and Hebrews would hang aloes on their doorways to protect the home from negative spirits and bring peace.

Honoring the four directions is an ancient practice used by civilizations around the world. Buddhism features a four-headed goddess that has a face looking in each of the four directions. The Judeo-Christian Bible features Ezekiel and his four-sided chariot, and the mystical teaching of kabbalah speaks of the four worlds. Native Americans pay homage to the four directions.

This ritual combines the peace-giving and lubricating essence of aloe with the long-held tradition of honoring the four directions.

This ritual can also be performed together by a couple in order to solidify their attraction. Each person rubs the aloe gel on the other, while saying the incantation together. This is a great warm-up for a passionate moon love session.

For this ritual you can use the inner gel from a live aloe vera plant, if you have one handy. Or you can get a tube of natural clear aloe vera gel from the health food store.

1 To attract a new lover, wait for the full moon, and go outside with a handful of crushed aloe vera in your left hand.

2 Toss pieces of the aloe with the right hand in each direction: north, west, south, and east.

3 After you toss the aloes north, rub the aloe gel between your eyes and say, "I see you, love, I see you come from the north." (If you have a particular person in mind, you can use his or her name instead of "love.")

4 Toss the aloes to the east, rub the aloe gel on your right nipple and say, "I see you, love, I see you come from the east."

5 Toss the aloes to the south. Rub the aloe gel on your genitals and say, "I see you, love, I see you come from the south."

6 Toss the aloes to the west. Rub the aloe gel on your left nipple and say, "I see you, love, I see you come from the west."

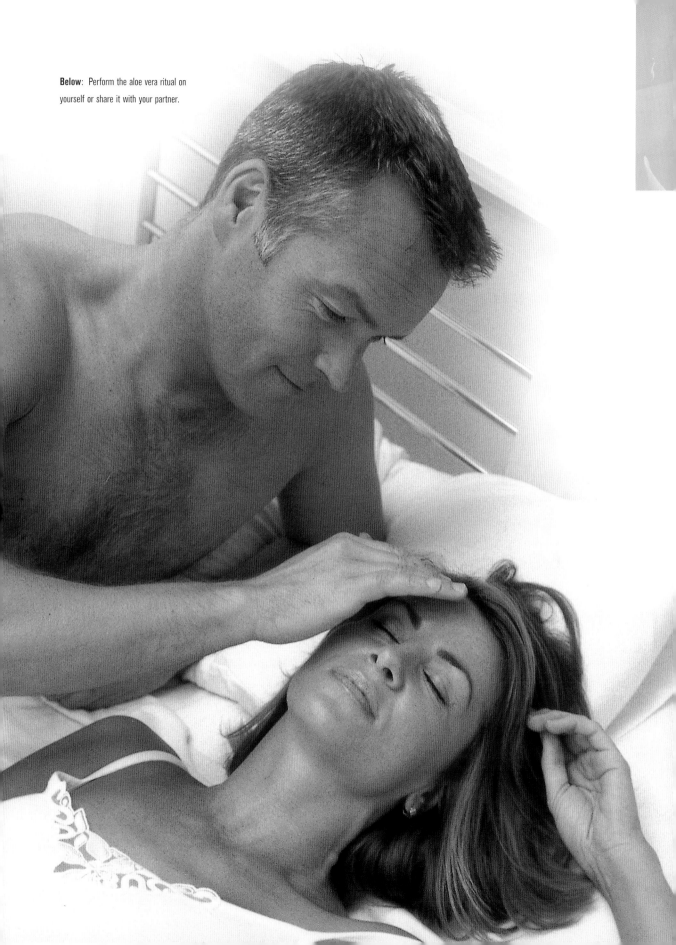

Below: Perform the aloe vera ritual on yourself or share it with your partner.

Water and Salt
Bathtime Bliss

Water is the most important element in the human body, making up 75 percent of our total structure and 85 percent of our brain. Water has always been the center of sacred rituals such as the Catholic baptism and the mikvah bath of the Hebrews used to signal a return to a sexual life after the cloistering during the menstrual flow. (Hence the presence of holy water in the entrance to temples.) Egyptians worshiped the Nile, and the Indians, the Ganges River.

A clear example of the importance of water to sexuality is illustrated by the Hindu god Vishnu. He is honored as the ruler of erotic feelings, as well as having the title Lord of the Waters. Water has also consistently been used to imply romance—think of the phrase "oceans of love." Sexuality and love relationships are often represented in literature by water images. Modern science is now documenting some remarkable attributes of water that have lent credence to its use since ancient times for its healing and virility-enhancing powers. Scientists have now found that water is capable of "storing" information. Its crystalline structure can be programmed and changed according to the energy surrounding it. The changed water can, in turn, influence those who come into contact with it (see Chapter 3, Energy-Based Remedies, for more information).

Salt is needed for every metabolic function in our body. The fluid that surrounds and is part of every cell contains salt. Many believe that the beginning of life in the salt waters of the sea is reflected in the salt content that we still float within. You have only to taste your own tears to experience the salinity of your inner fluids. Salt is a crystalline substance that has positive and negative polarity energy, which reflects the yin and yang attraction between lovers. The following ritual combines water and salt to produce a fluid, crystalline experience that can bring your love life to new heights.

Ingredients

Rainwater

Red candles and/or a red
    light bulb

Small bowl

Dead Sea salt, or coarse
    kosher salt

Damiana extract

Essential oils:
    Ylang ylang
    Vanilla
    Lavender

Almond massage oil

Instructions

1 Gather the rainwater beforehand. It can be kept for several months after gathering if necessary. Rainwater is considered "living water." It is believed by yogi teachers to be of a higher vibrational essence because it descends from the heavens.

2 Place red candles in the bathroom, or replace the bulb in the light fixture with a red bulb to enhance the erotic energy. Red stimulates the lower chakras involved in the sex response.

3 In a small bowl, place one cup of Dead Sea salt or coarse kosher salt.

4 Add a few tablespoons of the rainwater—just enough to moisten the salt, without dissolving it. Save the rest of the water on the side.

5 Add 30 drops of the damiana extract to the water and salt mixture. Damiana is a Mexican herb used as an aphrodisiac (see the section on herbs in Chapter 2 for more information).

6 Light the candles or turn on the red light, and start filling the bathtub with warm water.

7 While the water is running you and your lover stand with your feet in the bathtub.

8 Each partner takes turns picking up a handful of salt/herb mixture and uses it as a scrub on the other person. This takes off dead skin cells and creates a charge on the body, while the damiana further raises the sexual stimulation.

9 While performing the salt/herb rub, you can either say out loud, or quietly focus on, the following phrase: "I cleanse you, my beloved, we become one."

10 Use the salt/herb mixture on arms, elbows, legs, back, chest, and stomach, but do not get into eyes or sensitive vaginal tissues, because it can burn.

11 As the tub is filling, add five drops of each of the essential oils ylang ylang, vanilla, and lavender, and a tablespoon of almond massage oil. This will fill the room with a delicious erotic scent.

12 After completing the salt/herb scrub, both of you can sink down into the inviting water, facing each other (if the size of the bathtub allows), and allowing the oils to soothe your freshly exfoliated skin and your senses.

13 Breathe deeply in and out ten times in unison, while you gaze into each other's eyes, visualizing magnetic electrical energy passing through the water and engulfing both of you in a womblike resonant field.

14 Once you are both comfortable and relaxed, pour the remaining rainwater slowly over your partner's head. The contrast of the cool rainwater and the warm bath further awakens erotic energies.

15 Begin massaging each other, concentrating first on the feet, especially those points that relate to the sex organs (see the section on reflexology in Chapter 5 for more information).

16 Allow your imagination to run wild. The slippery texture of the oil, along with the buoyancy of the water, especially if you are in a large tub or spa, allows for experimentation with many new and varied positions. Enjoy!

Below: Bathing can be a highly erotic and healing experience–as well being fun!

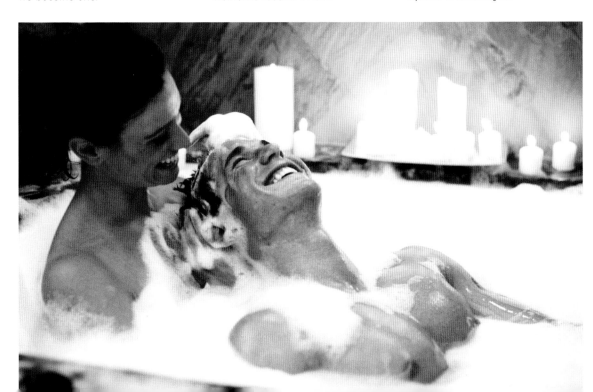

Amulet
Bags

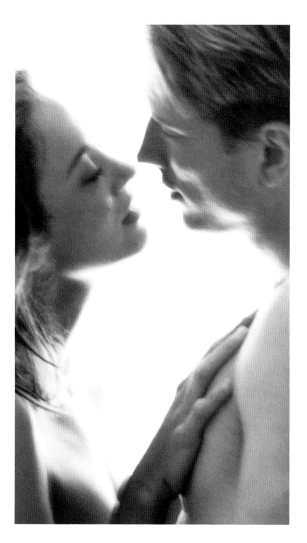

Above: You can use an amulet bag to increase sexual attraction.

The word *amulet* is derived from the Latin *amuletum,* which translates to "means of defense." Amulet bags have been called "conjure bags," "mojo," "hoodoo," and many other names in almost every human language that has ever existed. The amulet bag is made specifically to hold amulets—sacred objects that are believed to give special powers, such as protection against evil, or seducing money, luck, or love to the wearer. Every civilization from cave dwellers to modern cultures has had its own special amulets.

Amulets may be small carvings or statues that can fit into an amulet bag. In ancient Egypt, the frog amulet protected fertility. The Babylonians used a ram or bull amulet for virility, while in modern-day Thailand, penis amulets are popular. They are called *Palas khik,* which means "honorable surrogate penis." Perhaps the newest amulet is one made with a sample of your lover's DNA.

CHOOSE YOUR OWN INGREDIENTS

In addition to representational forms, many other items are used in amulet bags, such as herbs, gems, small pieces of paper with spells written on them, photos, or anything else that comes to mind. In magical circles, the teaching is that the best number of items in an amulet bag is 1 to 13, but the number should always be odd. Following are instructions for an amulet bag with nine items, particularly designed to increase sexual attraction.

You can use the recipe as a starter, then add four more of your own special amulets to individualize your amulet bag. Make one bag if it is only for you, or two if you want to share this with a lover.

Amulets are usually worn around the neck or pinned to underwear. Add a string if you wish to wear it around your neck. Share the amulet with your lover. Each of you can rub your amulet on your own genitals and those of your lover, allowing the sexual energy intention to imbibe into the amulet. You can then keep your amulet with you, and hold it and think of your lover when you want to psychically connect with him or her.

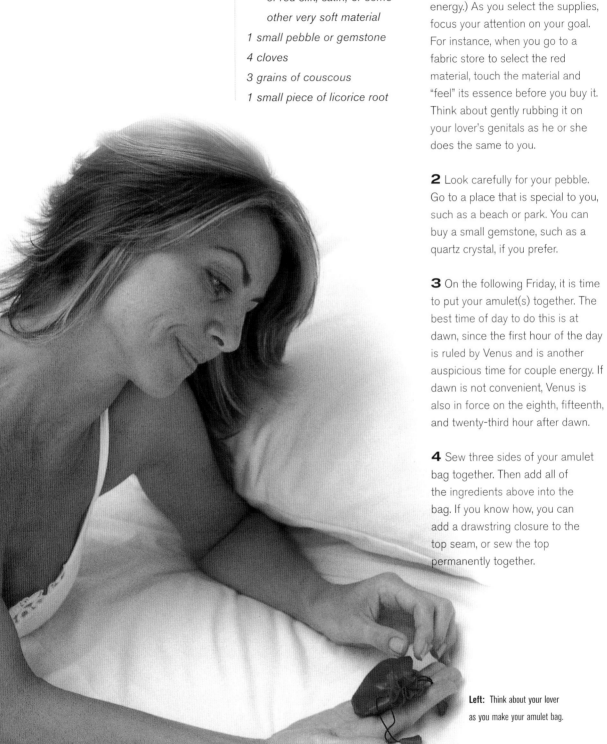

Supplies (for one bag):

*2 pieces measuring 2 inches
(5 cm) by 4 inches (10 cm)
of red silk, satin, or some
other very soft material*

1 small pebble or gemstone

4 cloves

3 grains of couscous

1 small piece of licorice root

1 Begin to shop for and gather your materials for your amulet bag on a Friday. (Friday is the day of the week most receptive to couple energy.) As you select the supplies, focus your attention on your goal. For instance, when you go to a fabric store to select the red material, touch the material and "feel" its essence before you buy it. Think about gently rubbing it on your lover's genitals as he or she does the same to you.

2 Look carefully for your pebble. Go to a place that is special to you, such as a beach or park. You can buy a small gemstone, such as a quartz crystal, if you prefer.

3 On the following Friday, it is time to put your amulet(s) together. The best time of day to do this is at dawn, since the first hour of the day is ruled by Venus and is another auspicious time for couple energy. If dawn is not convenient, Venus is also in force on the eighth, fifteenth, and twenty-third hour after dawn.

4 Sew three sides of your amulet bag together. Then add all of the ingredients above into the bag. If you know how, you can add a drawstring closure to the top seam, or sew the top permanently together.

Left: Think about your lover as you make your amulet bag.

103

7

CHAPTER SEVEN

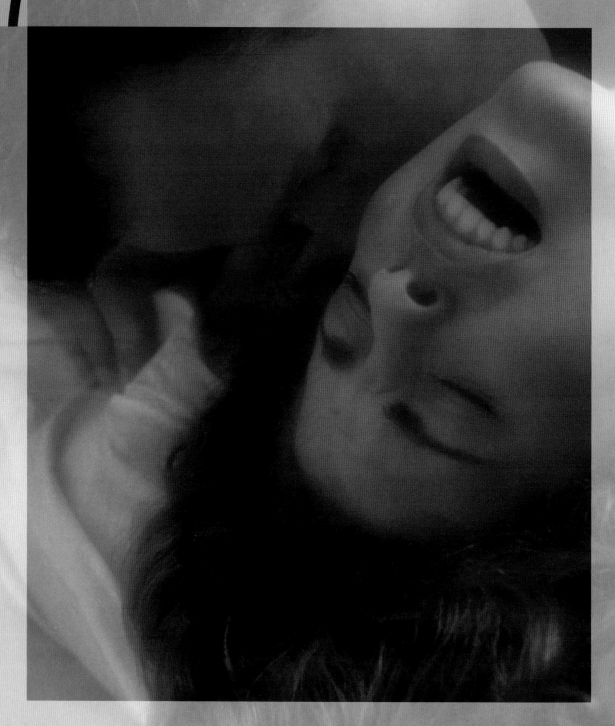

Orgasm is the ultimate culmination of the sexual experience. Although it is certainly not necessary to have an orgasm every time you make love, it is often the end goal. Orgasm has been studied by romantic poets, and intellectual scholars, and credible scientists, with all groups falling short of fully describing the experience. With this magical moment, it is really every man and woman for him/herself. Enjoy!

Orgasm— and Beyond

Ah, the orgasmic moment! The ultimate pleasure point may be one of life's most exquisite gifts. The word "orgasm" is derived from the Greek word *orgasmos*, which refers to lust, ripening, and swelling. A French expression for orgasm, "*la petite mort*," means "the little death," in reference to the feeling that one loses oneself in ecstasy.

When we work toward improving the quality of the orgasm, there is an almost opposite focal point for men and women. In men, there is an effort to forestall climaxing by maintaining an erection and avoiding premature ejaculation in order to extend the lovemaking session. Although most men regularly achieve orgasm, this innate ability may be interfered with by many kinds of prescription drugs, as well as physical ailments. Psychologically, men may feel pressure to ensure that their partner is satisfied. This concern can have the reverse effect and be a large part of the cause of their inability to perform.

For a woman, achieving orgasm is much less of a certainty. According to research, up to 15 percent of women have never achieved orgasm. About 25 percent claim that masturbation is the only way they are successful. Inability to achieve orgasm in both men and women may be due to psychological factors such as sexual abuse or a negative sexual experience, which can leave a lifelong scar that inhibits the orgasmic response.

Counseling may help, because the more open, honest, and comfortable a person feels about sex, the more likely he or she is to experience orgasm. Along with the body–mind connection, improved nutrition, daily exercise, and stress reduction techniques can all aid in achieving a consistent and successful orgasmic response.

Orgasms vary in intensity. The earth doesn't always move! This difference can usually be attributed to psychological factors, such as the state of relaxed loving feelings between the participants. A "quickie" performed out of a sense of duty at the end of a stressful day will yield a different climax than a romantic evening complete with a sensuous dinner, luxurious bath, soft music, exotic lingerie, candlelight, pleasant aromas, and silk sheets.

Orgasmic "Apparatus":
The Clitoris and the Penis

The clitoris is a remarkable organ. It is the only structure known that has no other function than to provide sexual pleasure. The penis seconds as a urinary passageway, while the vagina is also a birth canal, but the clitoris is unique as a stand-alone "love button." It is fascinating to contemplate how this pleasure-only organ evolved, especially since it is not necessary for a woman to be brought to orgasm in order to conceive. On the other hand, outside of interventions such as artificial insemination, male ejaculation through orgasm *is* needed to bring about the blessed event.

In most women, direct stimulation of the area surrounding the clitoris is necessary to achieve orgasm, although there are exceptions, such as women who say that they have orgasms during "doggie-style" penetration. The kind of stroking, timing, and the amount of pressure needed to achieve orgasm varies greatly from one woman to another. Many women who claim to be able to reach orgasm only through masturbation are probably successful because they are in total control of these clitoral stimulation parameters. Lubrication of the clitoris repeatedly during sexual play, along with maintaining clitoral contact during intercourse through correct positioning, will help to trigger orgasm during intercourse. The ability to totally relax and let go is necessary, too. Trying hard to achieve a climax can have an inhibiting effect. Many women report that

they have better orgasms as they age—especially into their 30s and 40s, as they become more secure and attain a more relaxed attitude and a higher level of self-esteem.

The clitoris and the penis have some structural parameters in common. The rounded tip of both organs is called the "glans," the only part of the clitoris that is visible in most women. The elongated shaft of the clitoris is approximately 1 to 3 inches (25–76 mm), with two arms, or *crura,* that run under the muscles below both sides of the lips of the vagina. The clitoral muscles contract due to nerves that travel throughout the pelvic region, along the vagina, urethra, and bladder. Similar to the penis, the clitoris contains erectile spongy tissue that becomes engorged with blood and doubles in size when aroused. This can occur due to tactile stimulation to the genital area, breasts, thighs, other erogenous zones, or even sexy thoughts. Most woman find that direct stimulation to the clitoris when it is aroused is too intense and may even feel annoying or painful. Soft stimulation or pressure on the surrounding area is usually preferred.

The debate over whether there is a difference between vaginal and clitoral orgasms has raged since the time of Freud. Although scientific studies have determined that all female orgasms are initiated via the clitoris, many women claim that they experience a difference, with some orgasms feeling like they are centered around the clitoris, while at other times, the experience floods into the vaginal walls and even the anal sphincter muscles.

The penis has three parts: the root, which attaches to the lower trunk of the body, the elongated shaft, and the glans, or rounded head. The penis is covered with loose skin, called the foreskin, which is removed if the man has been circumcised. The frenulum is the area on the underside of the penis where the foreskin is attached to the head. It is sometimes referred to as the male clitoris, because it is an ultrasensitive area that is richly supplied with nerve endings. If the foreskin is intact, it will slide over the frenulum during sex. In a circumcised man, stimulation to this area with a little extra pressure will often initiate an orgasm. The spongy tissue inside the penis becomes engorged with blood when a man becomes sexually aroused; this causes an erection. The size of the flaccid penis may not be indicative of the size of the same penis when it is erect. The penis, like the clitoris, is an incredible organ, and is worshipped as an icon in several Eastern sects.

LUBRICATION

For sex to be enjoyable, lubrication is necessary. The vagina (and the penis, in some men) begins to release natural lubricants in the early stages of sexual arousal. However, the amount of lubrication varies from person to person, and from one sexual encounter to another in the same person. Most people will want to have additional lubrication handy during sex. Saliva works as a great sexual lubricant, as long as there is no risk of infection.

There are many water-based commercial lubricants available on the market. Try several different brands; some dry quickly and have to be continuously reapplied. Always use a water-based, rather than an oil-based, lubricant if condoms are being used, because oil can cause the latex condom to break down. Oil-based lubricants can be very satisfying, however, if they are all natural, organic, and edible. Pure Vitamin E oil, almond oil, or sesame oil works well.

Below: Feeling relaxed is important when trying to achieve orgasm.

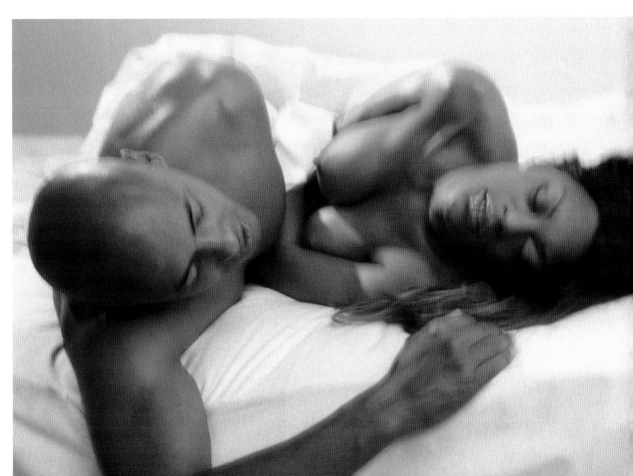

Sexual Response Cycle:
Excitement, Plateau, Orgasm, Recovery

Men and woman experience the same four phases in the sexual response cycle, but each person has his or her own unique variation in terms of timing in moving through each phase. Learn to consider these differences, and consciously adjust your own transition from one cycle to the other to accommodate your partner. It is not necessary for the timing to be exactly the same and, in fact, this is rarely the case. Occasionally, both partners experience orgasm simultaneously. Although this is extremely enjoyable to both parties, it is usually a happy coincidence.

Excitement

The excitement phase occurs during the initiation of the sexual encounter. In couples who have been lovers over a period of time, the excitement phase may last only a few minutes. The physical effects include the beginning of blood flow to the genitals, which causes a swelling, reddening, and increase in size in both sexes. At this point, vaginal lubrication will usually occur, as well as hardening of the nipples. The skin may become flushed or blotched, and some men also begin to secrete a lubricating fluid.

Below: Stages of a female orgasm. Excitement rises to a peak during climax and creates a series of peak experiences over subsequent orgasms.

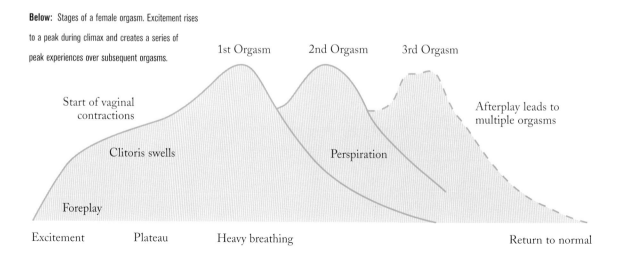

Start of vaginal contractions

1st Orgasm   2nd Orgasm   3rd Orgasm

Afterplay leads to multiple orgasms

Clitoris swells   Perspiration

Foreplay

Excitement   Plateau   Heavy breathing   Return to normal

Plateau

All the changes in the excitement phase continue to intensify. The plateau phase lasts until just before the orgasmic release, so the time can vary extensively. Muscle spasms may occur in the hands, feet, and face; hence the expression "He/she makes my toes curl." Blood pressure increases; heart rates and breathing become heavier.

Orgasm

At the point of orgasm, breathing is rapid and there is a sudden release of sexual tension. In men, the base of the penis begins rhythmic contractions causing the ejaculation of semen. Women experience orgasm as a rhythmic sequence of vaginal contractions that may also spread to the uterus. Orgasm usually lasts for four to twenty seconds. Many people vocalize with loud grunts, screams, or other sounds, and may get a rashlike sex flush on the skin.

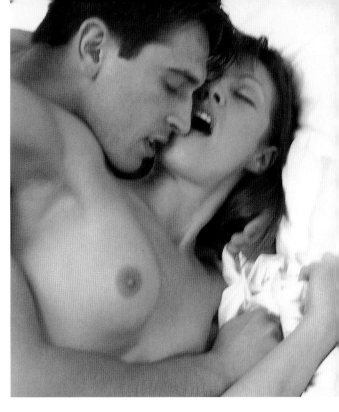

Above: At the point of orgasm, sexual tension is released.

Recovery

Following orgasm, the breathing, blood pressure, and heart rate return to normal, and blood drains from the genitals. Many women can recover quickly, and go on to have several more multiple orgasms, if stimulation continues beyond the first peak. Men have a more sharply defined "road to release." Once they climax and ejaculate, they usually cannot have a second orgasm for a longer recovery time. Young men might need as little as one-half to one hour, but twelve to twenty-four hours is a more usual cycle in mature men. During the recovery phase most people experience an afterglow where cuddling, synchronous breathing, and feelings of relaxation and well-being are common.

Below: Stages leading to male orgasm. There is a steep increase in sexual excitement during early foreplay. This levels off and then rises again as the man reaches ejaculation.

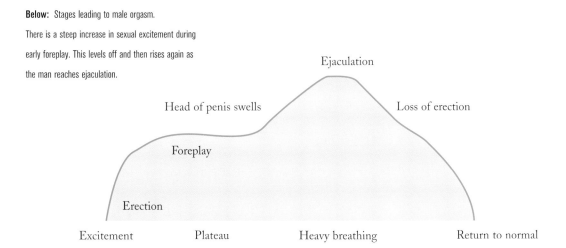

Sex on Your Own:
Masturbation

There are many reasons why an individual would indulge in "single sex." We don't all have sex partners available at all times. Many people enjoy masturbation and other forms of self-stimulation, and may find they are able to reach a more intense climax alone than with a partner; this is especially true for women. Research indicates that masturbation is a widespread practice with 95 percent of men and 89 percent of women reporting that they have masturbated. Old taboos have included the belief that masturbation is a harmful form of self-abuse that indicates a mental imbalance and could cause disease and skin disorders, such as acne. These beliefs are unfounded. Modern research has shown that masturbation can be a therapeutic technique that helps increase self-confidence and the ability to share sexually with others.

MALE ENERGY

According to the Eastern traditions of Tao and tantra, masturbation, along with any sexual act, has deep connections to the emotional and spiritual aspects of the soul, as well as providing physical gratification. Male masturbation that ends in orgasm is believed to decrease the overall life-force energy, which is held in the semen. If sex is shared with a woman, the essential feminine essence can help to regenerate the male energy, but solitary sex does not provide for the regenerative sharing. Therefore, these teachings suggest that if a man indulges in single sex, he should stop short of ejaculation, and use visualization and breathing techniques (as described in Circulating Chi in Chapter 3) to circulate the sexual charge he has built up through self-stimulation in order to energize and regenerate his internal organs. If semen is ejaculated, the ancients suggested that it be used for a sacred ritual purpose, such as adding it to amulet bags (see

Below: Male masturbation that ends in orgasm is believed to reduce overall energy.

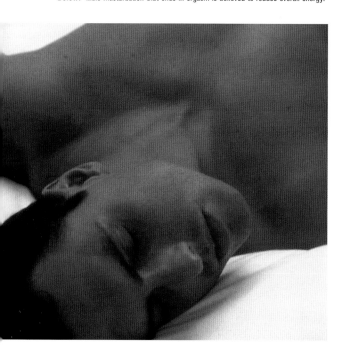

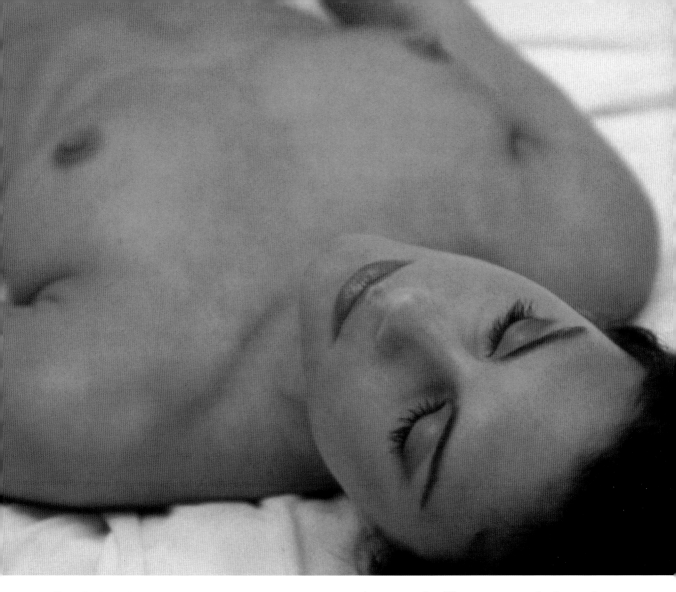

Above: Female masturbation is thought to enhance overall energy.

the section "Amulet Bags" earlier in this chapter) or burying it in the garden to energize the land.

FEMALE ENERGY

Women, however, are thought to have boundless stores of sexual energy that is enhanced by self-stimulation ending in one or multiple orgasms. A woman is encouraged to satisfy her sexuality at will, with any number of stimulatory techniques. Erotic daydreams are believed to help build sexual energy, which can be released with or without the use of a substitute phallus (such as a dildo) or a phallic-shaped fruit or vegetable such as a cucumber. The woman can make the experience more meaningful for her spiritual self by focusing on higher-level thoughts at the time of orgasm, and by circulating the orgasmic energy up her spine to her brain and other internal organs.

A common practice in Eastern societies was to have an exact replica of a husband's penis made from a smooth hard substance, such as jade or wood, that a woman could use as a masturbation device when her lover was absent. The use of sex toys continues to be popular in modern times, with a large variety of dildos, vibrators, and other stimulating devices widely available. You can find a selection of suppliers in the Resources section on page 122.

Orgasm—and Beyond

The Female
G–spot

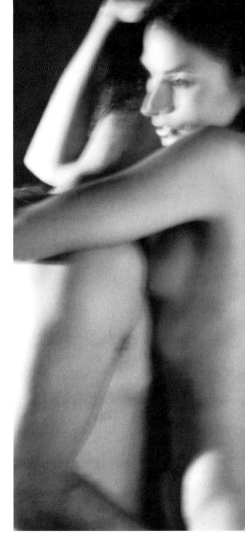

Above: Find the G-spot for multiple orgasms.

The G-spot was named after Dr. Ernest Grafenberg, who is credited with "discovering" this somewhat remote supersensitive sexual zone, which he described in a paper published in 1950. Called the "sacred spot" for centuries in Eastern teachings, this area of the woman's anatomy has to be searched for. It can usually be located in the middle of the upper front wall of the vagina right behind the pubic bone. The area surrounding the G-Spot is spongy erectile tissue that becomes swollen when stimulated.

Women have a variety of reactions to G-spot play. Many women claim that stimulating the G-spot is the surest route to the bliss of multiple orgasms. Most women are totally satisfied with their single climax, and should never feel compelled to have several orgasms in a row in order to feel completed. If you do choose to "go for the gold," after reaching the first climax, don't stop the stimulation. Keep the pressure on, and lubricate again if needed. It may help to increase the intensity of the stimulation until you experience another buildup of energy.

The feeling has been described as a "pyramid effect," with an increase in intensity as you move from the first orgasmic climax to the next. In order to achieve this, it may help to increase the intensity of the stimulation until you experience another buildup of energy. Many women claim that the doggie-style position puts just the right kind of pressure on the G-spot. Others actually "ejaculate" a sweet, clear fluid that is not urine, but similar to male ejaculate without the sperm. Then again, not everyone enjoys stimulation of the G-spot; some claim that it is painful or annoying. A common reaction is to feel the urge to urinate, although this feeling may disappear with continued stimulation. It may work best for a woman to try it herself and then explain to her lover the best technique to bring her to G-spot heaven.

To find the G-spot, do the following exercise.

1 Insert well-lubricated fingers about 2 inches (50 mm) into the vagina.

2 Bend the fingers up toward the navel.

3 Press against the top of the front wall of the vagina and see if you can feel an area that feels somewhat spongy.

4 Rub gently back and forth around this area. It will often start to become erect and sensitive.

The Male
G-spot

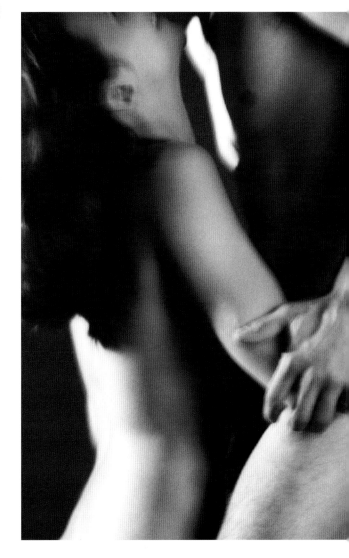

Although there is no actual G-spot in men, there is an area that is analogous to the female G-spot. It has been referred to as the Million Dollar Point in Oriental traditions. No man (or woman) should feel that finding this elusive trigger point is compulsory for sexual enjoyment. If you choose to do so, approach your search as you would an exciting adventure.

The area is located along the midline of the lower part of the body, between the anus and the testicles. Probe around the area, until you find a small indentation. Stimulate by pushing inward, gently, in a circular motion.

Another way to access the male G-spot is through internal stimulation. Many people prefer to use a latex glove to try this. First lubricate the gloved finger. Then slowly insert the finger, checking that it does not cause any pain. Go at a snail's pace, since the outer third of the rectum is the most sensitive and many claim stimulating this area is the most enjoyable sensation.

Once everyone is relaxed sufficiently, insert the finger more deeply, curl the finger upward, in a "come hither" motion and tap the prostate and the area of bone behind it.

Some men have an intense orgasm following this, while others tend to lose their erection, and some men do not enjoy the feeling.

Right: Stimulating the male G-spot can intensify a man's orgasm.

Sex
after 60

There is a host of evidence supporting the fact that human sexuality is not strictly a mechanism for survival of the species. Humans enjoy and employ sexual activities at all times, not only when the body is in a fertile state. Sexuality can continue into advanced age, long past the possibility of reproduction. Many people who have entered the "golden years" say that they are having the best sex yet! Gone are the days of concern over unwanted pregnancy. Also, people who are retired have more relaxation time. They can loll around in bed late in the morning if they so choose, and don't have as many responsibilities and interruptions.

A study analyzed women who had already gone through menopause and found that, while frequency of sexual encounters decreased somewhat with age, enjoyment and satisfaction associated with sex was just as high as in younger women.[1] In a very real sense, the old adage "If you don't use it, you lose it," applies to sexual function. Women who continue to experience sexual stimulation, either with a partner or by masturbating, have less thinning and drying of the vagina after menopause.[2]

As men age, they enter "andropause," which has many similarities to menopause in woman, including a decrease in sex hormones. This can slow the sexual response in men and increase the time it takes to get an erection, although it does not have to dampen the pleasure. Many men report that they actually enjoy sex more because they are more relaxed, take their time, and are not as goal-oriented in terms of achieving an orgasm.

Research indicates that older women are actually more interested in sex than older men. Perhaps this is because women are more involved with the love and emotional aspects of sex, while men are more connected to lust and the ability to orgasm, which reduces with age. Seniors who regularly engage in sex have a higher level of overall physical and mental health than their abstinent counterparts. Sexually active people have a higher level of self-esteem, a better body image, and a greater feeling of emotional connection than those who don't indulge. Even long-term partners often find a whole new level of romantic involvement in the later years. Once the children are gone and work duties have disappeared, many couples claim it is "like meeting all over again." They remember what attracted them to their partner in the first place, which may have been lost in the busy years of career and family.

In both men and women, efforts to strive for maximum health and wellness through daily exercise, nutritious eating, the therapeutic use of herbs and nutrients, as well as spiritual pursuits, enhance all of life's pleasures, including extending sexual function well into the golden years!

Right: Evidence shows that age need not be a block to sexual enjoyment.

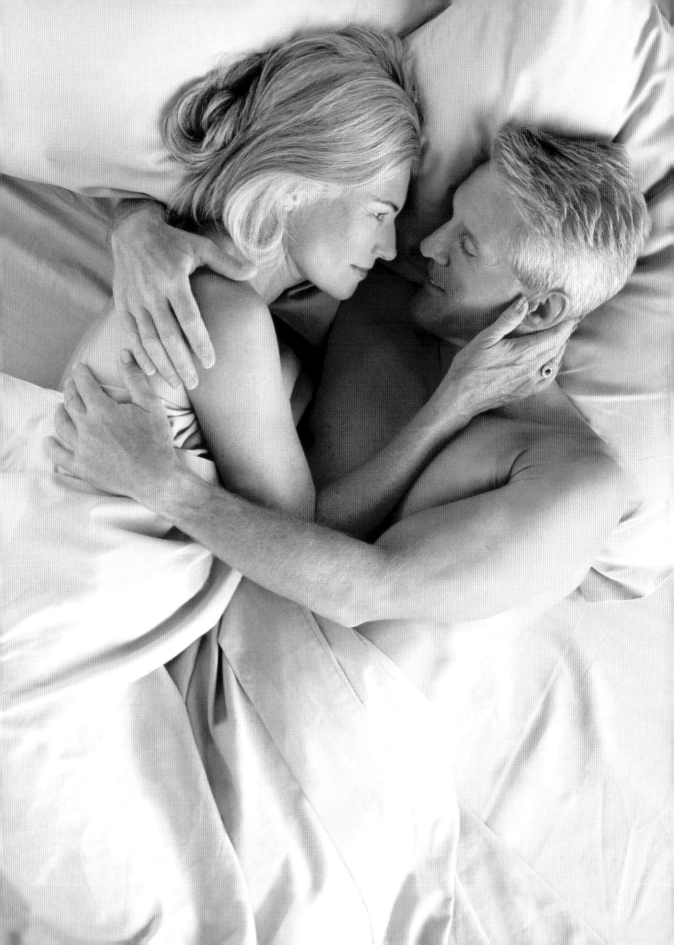

Notes

INTRODUCTION

1. Dolphins are also reported to engage in bisexual activity regularly, not only during fertile seasons.

CHAPTER ONE

1. The topic of Natural Hormone Replacement is discussed in depth in the author's book *Cycles of Life*, pp. 1–6.

2. L. Hackbert, J. R. Heiman, "Acute dehydroepiandrosterone (DHEA) effects on sexual arousal in postmenopausal women," *Journal of Women's Health and Gender-Based Medicine*, March 2002, 11(2): 155–62.

3. C. E. Dean, "Prasterone (DHEA) and mania," *Annals of Pharmacotherapy*, December 2000, 34(12): 1419–22.

4. C. M. Meston, P.F. Frohlich, "The neurobiology of sexual function," *Archives of General Psychiatry*, May 2002, 59(5): 469–70.

CHAPTER TWO

1. B. Hong, Y. H. Ji, J .H. Hong, K. Y. Nam, T. Y. Ahn, "A double-blind crossover study evaluating the efficacy of Korean red ginseng in patients with erectile dysfunction: a preliminary report," *Journal of Urology*, Nov 2002, 168(5): 2027–33.

2. Xiao Yong Xin, "A Pharmacological Study of Wu Zi Zhuang Yang Tang," Part 1, *Journal of Pharmacology and Clinical Practice of Traditional Chinese Medicine*, 1989, 5(2): 21. Also Part II, 5(5): 34.

3. G. J. Park, S. P. Mann, M. C. Ngu, "Acute hepatitis induced by Shou-Wu-Pian, a herbal product derived from polygonum multiflorum," *Journal of Gastroenterol Hepatology*, 2001 Jan, 16(1): 115–7.

4. A. L. da Silva, S. Bardini, S. S. Nunes, E. Elisabetsky, "Anxiogenic properties of Ptychopetalum olacoides Benth (Marapuama)," *Phytotherapy Research*, 2002 May, 16(3): 223–6.

5. E. Ernst, M. H. Pittler, "Yohimbine for erectile dysfunction: A systematic review and meta-analysis of randomized clinical trials," *Journal of Urology*, 1998, 159: 433–6.

6. Robert H. Fletcher, Kathleen Fairfield, "Vitamins for Chronic Disease Prevention in Adults," *Journal of the American Medical Association*, 2002, 287: 3127.

7. M. Scibona, et al., "L-arginine and Male Infertility," *Minerva Urologica Nefrologica*, Dec 1994, 46(4): 251-3.

8. C. M. Meston, M. Worcel, "The effects of yohimbine plus L-arginine glutamate on sexual arousal in postmenopausal women with sexual arousal disorder," *Archives of Sexual Behavior*, Aug 2002, 31(4): 323–32.

9. S. Thys-Jacobs, P. Starkey, D. Bernstein, et al. "Calcium carbonate and the premenstrual syndrome: Effects on premenstrual and menstrual symptoms," *American Journal of Obstetrics and Gynecology*, 1998, 179: 444–52.

CHAPTER THREE

1. J. R. White, D. A. Case, D. McWhirter, A. M. Mattison, "Enhanced sexual behavior in exercising men," *Urology*, 55(4): 598–602.

CHAPTER FOUR

1. Wilhelm Reich, M.D., "Experimental Investigation of the Electrical Function of Sexuality and Anxiety," *The Journal of Orgonomy*, 3, 1969, (1 & 2).

CHAPTER FIVE

1. J. H Hagemann, G. Berding, S. Bergh, et al., "Effects of

Visual Sexual Stimuli and Apomorphine SL on Cerebral Activity in Men with Erectile Dysfunction," *European Urology* Apr 2003; 43(4): 412–20.

2. K. A. Wientjes, "Mind-body techniques in wound healing," *Ostomy Wound Management,* 2002, Nov 48, (11): 62–7.

3. V. W. Donaldson, "A clinical study of visualization on depressed white blood cell count in medical patients," *Applied Psychophysiology Biofeedback* 2000, Jun, 25(2): 117–28.

4. C. Lorch, V. Lorch, A. Diefendors, et al., "Effects of Stimulative and Sedative Music on Systolic Blood Pressure, Heart Rate and Respiratory Rate in Premature Infants," *Journal of Music Therapy*, 1994, 31(2): 108–18.

5. B. Bittman, L. Berk, D. Selton, et al., "Composite Effects of Group Drumming Music Therapy on Modulation of Neuroendocrine–Immune Parameters in Normal Subjects," *Alternative Therapies*, Jan 2001.

6. Darwin, Charles, *The Descent of Man and Selection in Relation to Sex*, (1871), John Murray Publishers, London, UK, p. 880.

7. Miller, Geoffrey F, (2000) Evolution of Music Through Sexual Selection, in *The Origins Of Music*, N.L.Wallin, B. Merker, and S. Brown (editors), Center for Economic Learning and Social Evolution, University College, London, England, MIT Press, pp. 329–360.

8. S. Alt-Epping, T. Ostermann, J. Schmidt, "Diagnosis of appendicitis with particular consideration of the acupuncture point Lanwei—a prospective study," *Forsch Komplementarmed Klass Naturheilkd,* Dec 2002, 9(6): 338–450.

9. L. S. Yaman, S. Kilic, K. Sarica, et, al., "The place of acupuncture in the management of psychogenic impotence," *European Urology*, 1994, 26(1): 52–5.

10. Kathleen Stern, Martha K. McClintock, *Nature* 392, 177–179 (12 Mar 1998).

CHAPTER SEVEN

1. K. Hawton, D. Gath, A. Day, "Sexual function in a community sample of middle-aged women with partners: effects of age, marital, socioeconomic, psychiatric, gynecological, and menopausal factors," *Archives of Sexual Behavior,* Aug 1994, 23(4): 375–95.

2. M. K. Beard, "Atrophic vaginitis. Can it be prevented?" *Post Graduate Medicine* May 1992, 91: 257.

Bibliography

Amini, Fari, Thomas Lewis, and Richard Lannon.
A General Theory of Love.
New York: Random House, 1999.

Anand, Margo. *The Art of Sexual Magic.*
New York: Jeremy Tarcher, 1995.

Beattie, Antonia. *Love Magic.*
New York: Barnes and Noble Books, 2000.

Cerney, J. V. *Acupuncture without Needles.*
New York: Parker Publishing, 1974.

Chia, Mantak. *Taoist Secrets of Love, Cultivating Male Sexual Energy.*
Santa Fe: Aurora Press, 1984.

—— *Healing Love through the Tao: Cultivating Male Sexual Energy.*
Huntington: Healing Tao Books, 1986.

—— *The Multi-Orgasmic Man.*
San Francisco: Harper Publishers, 2000.

Danielou, Alain. *The Hindu Temple.*
Rochester: Inner Traditions, 2001.

Douglas, Nik and Penny Slinger. *Sexual Secrets.*
Rochester: Destiny Books, 2000.

Dubitsky, Carl. *Bodywork Shiatsu.*
Rochester: Healing Arts Press, 1997.

Dunas, Felice. *Passion Play.* New York:
Riverhead Books, 1997.

Evola, Julius. *The Yoga of Power: Tantra, Shakti and The Secret Way.*
Rochester: Inner Traditions, 1992.

Ferguson, Pamela. *The Self-Shiatsu Handbook.*
New York: Berkley Publishing, 1995.

Gray, John. *Mars and Venus in the Bedroom.*
New York: Harper Collins, 1995.

Green, James. *The Male Herbal.*
Freedom: Crossing Press, 1991.

Jensen, Bernard. *Love, Sex and Nutrition.*
Garden City: Avery Publishing, 1988.

Petro Roybal, Beth Ann and Gayle Skowronski. *Sexy Up.*
Berkeley: Ulysses Press, 2002.

Kamhi, Ellen. *Cycles of Life, Herbs for Women.*
New York: M. Evans, 2001.

Lorenzo, Rafael. *A Sacred Sex Devotional.*
Rochester: Inner Traditions, 2000.

Mars, Brigitte. *Sex, Love and Health.*
North Bergen: Basic Health Publications, 2002.

Miller, Richard A., *The Magical and Ritual Use of Herbs,*
Seattle: Oak Press, 1977.

—— *The Magical and Ritual Use of Aphrodisiacs,* New York: Destiny Books, 1985.

Miller, Richard and Iona. *The Magical and Ritual Use of Perfumes,* New York: Destiny Books, 1990.

—— *The Modern Alchemist,* Grand Rapids: Phanes Press, 1994.

Oumano, Elena. *Natural Sex.* New York: Penguin Group Publishers, 1999.

Ramsdale, David and Ellen Ramsdale. *Lovemaking Secrets of the East and West.* New York: Bantam Doubleday Dell, 1993.

Reichenberg-Ullman, Judyth. *Whole Woman Homeopathy.* Roseville: Prima Health, 2000.

Riva, Anna. *The Modern Herbal Spellbook.* Toluca Lake: International Imports, 1974.

Sachs, Robert. *The Passionate Buddha, Wisdom on Intimacy and Enduring Love.* Rochester: Inner Traditions, 2002.

Shealy, C. Norman. *Miracles Do Happen.* Shaftesbury, Dorset: Element Books, 1995.

Stubbs, Kenneth Ray. New York: Secret Garden Publishers, 1992.

—— *Secret Sexual Positions: Ancient Techniques for Modern Lovers.* New York: Jeremy Tarcher, 1999.

Tisserand, Maggie. *Aromatherapy for Women.* Rochester: Healing Arts Press, 1996.

Weed, Susan. *New Menopausal Years.* Woodstock: Ash Tree Publishing, 2002.

Winkler, Gershon. *Sacred Secrets, The Sanctity of Sex in Jewish Law and Lore.* Northvale: Jason Aronson, Inc., 1998.

Yudelove, Eric. *The Tao and the Tree of Life.* Saint Paul: Llewellyn Publishers, 1995.

Zampieron, Eugene and Ellen Kamhi. *The Natural Medicine Chest.* Oyster Bay: Natural Alternatives, 2002.

Resources

APHRODISIAC FOODS

This site has a great selection of aphrodisiac recipes.

GourmetSleuth.com

P.O. Box 508

Los Gatos, California

Phone: 408-354-8281

Fax: 408-395-8279

Web: *http://www.gourmetsleuth.com/recipes_aphro.asp*

COMPOUNDING PHARMACIES

Compounding pharmacies prepare prescription drugs "made to order" for the individual according to a physician's order. To find a compounding pharmacy in your area, you can contact:

The International Academy of Compounding

Pharmacists (IACP)

P.O. Box 1365

Sugar Land, Texas 77487

Phone: 281-933-8400, 800-927-4227

Fax: 281-495-0602

E-mail: *iacpinfo@iacprx.org*

ESSENCE REMEDIES

Bach Flower Remedies prepared according to the instructions of Dr Edward Bach:

Dr. Edward Bach Centre

Mount Vernon, Bakers Lane

Sotwell, Oxon, OX10 0PZ,

United Kingdom

Phone: +44 (0) 1491 834678

Fax: +44 (0) 1491 825022

Web: *http://www.bachcentre.com*

Himalayan remedies prepared by Drs. Rupa and Atul Shah. Made from water from the Ganges River and flowers from the Himalayas.

Aum Himalaya Sanjeevini Essences

15 Em Jai Bharat Society, Third Road, Khar West

Mumbai (Bombay)—400 052, India

Tel. 648 68 19/604 75 29

Fax: (00-91-22) 605 09 75

E-mail: *rupaatul@bom3.vsnl.net.in*

Web: *www.aumhimalaya.com*

Perelandra remedies prepared by Machelle Small Wright from plants grown at the Perelandra Gardens.

Perelandra Gardens

P.O. Box 3603

Warrenton, Virginia 20188

U.S. and Canada Order Line: 1-800-960-8806

Overseas or Mexico Order Line: 1-540-937-2153

Fax: 1-540-937-3360

E-mail: *email@perelandra-ltd.com*

Web: *http://www.perelandra-ltd.com*

Prepares North American flower essences.

Flower Essence Services

P.O. Box 1769

Nevada City, California 95959

Phone: 800-548-0075, 530-265-0258

Fax: 530-265-6467

E-mail: *info@fesflowers.com*

Web: *http://www.fesflowers.com*

Tools for personal empowerment—flower essences, gems, and more.

Rainbow Resources

Web: *http://www.rainbowcrystal.com/bach/calif2.html#pers*

A unique line of skin products that combine the power of crystals, the dynamics of color, and the known benefits of essential oils.

Gematherapy

Phone: 615-354-1400

Email: *Gematherapy@aol.com*

Web: *http://www.gematherapy.com*

High-quality essential oils.
Original Swiss Aromatics,
P.O. Box 6842
San Rafael, California 94903
Phone: 415-479-9120
Fax: 415-479-0614
Web: *http://www.originalswissaromatics.com*

High-quality essential oils and tantric workshops.
Vedic Harmonics Essential Oils
P.O. Box 35284
Sarasota, California 34242
Phone: 800-370-3220
Web: *http://www.ayurvedichealers.com*

HERBALISTS
American Herbalist's Guild
1931 Gaddis Road
Canton, Georgia 30115
Phone: 770-751-6021
Fax: 770-751-7472
E-mail: ahgoffice@earthlink.net
Web: *http://www.americanherbalist.com*

American Botanical Council
P.O. Box 14345
Austin, Texas 78714-4345
Phone: 800-373-7105, 512- 331-8868
Web: *http://www.herbalgram.org*

HERB SOURCES
Growers and providers of fresh and dried organic bulk herbs, medicinal plants, and other herbal products.
Frontier Natural Products Co-op
P.O. Box 299
3021 78th Street
Norway, Iowa 52318
Phone: 800-669-3275, 319-227-7996
Fax: 319-227-7966
E-mail: *customercare@frontiercoop.com*
Web: *http://www.frontiercoop.com*

Horizon Herbs
P.O. Box 69
Williams, Oregon 97544
Phone: 541-846-6704
Fax: 541-846-6233
E-mail: *hhcustserv@HorizonHerbs.com*
Web: *http://www.chatlink.com/~herbseed/*

Nature's Answer
75 Commerce Avenue
Hauppauge, New York 11788
Phone: 800-439-2324
Web: *http://www.naturesanswer.com*

HOMEOPATHY
Education and information about homeopathy.
The National Center for Homeopathy
801 North Fairfax Street, Suite 306
Alexandria, Virginia 22314
Phone: 703-548-7790
Web: *http://www.homeopathic.org*

ABC Homeopathy
This web site offers a complete on-line information service about homeopathy, including a comprehensive symptom-based remedy locator.
Web: *http://www.abchomeopathy.com*

School of Homeopathy
Homeopathic Training
Orchard House, Merthyr Road
Llanfoist NP7 9LN
United Kingdom
Phone: (+44/0)1873-856872
Fax: (+44/0)1873-858962
E-mail: *stuart@homeopathyschool.com*

The National Center for Homeopathy
801 North Fairfax Street, Suite 306
Alexandria, Virginia 22314
Phone: 703-548-7790
Web: *http://www.homeopathic.org*

KABBALAH

The Kabbalah Center
155 E. 48th Street
New York, New York 10017
Phone: 212-644-0025
Fax: 212-644-0634
Web: *http://www.kabbalah.com*

NATURAL ALTERNATIVES HEALTH, EDUCATION, AND MULTIMEDIA SERVICES

P.O. Box 525
Oyster Bay, New York 11771
Phone: 800-829-0918
E-mail: *naturalalt@juno.com*
Web: *http://www.naturalnurse.com*

NATURAL ALTERNATIVES HERBAL WORKSHOPS

with Ellen Kamhi, The Natural Nurse, and Eugene Zampieron, N.D.
Call for updated schedule
Phone: 800-829-0918
Web: *http://www.naturalnurse.com*

ORGONE ENERGY

Information and courses about the life and work of Wilhelm Reich and orgone energy.
The American College of Orgonomy
P.O. Box 490
Princeton, New Jersey 08542
Phone: 732-821-1144
Fax: 732-821-0174
E-mail: *aco@orgonomy.org*
Web: *http://www.orgonomy.org*

SALIVA TESTING

Used to determine hormone levels. In some areas individuals can order the test for themselves. Other geographic areas require a physician's order.
Aeron LifeCycles Clinical Laboratory
1933 Davis Street, Suite 310

San Leandro, California 94577
Phone: 800-631-7900
Fax: 510-729-0383
E-mail: *aeron@aeron.com*
Web: *http://www.aeron.com*

SEX EDUCATION AND THERAPY

Information about certified sex therapists.
American Association of Sex Educators, Counselors and Therapists
P.O. Box 5488
Richmond, Virginia 23220-0488
Web: *http://www.aasect.org*

A graduate program in the study of human sexuality.
Institute for the Advanced Study of Human Sexuality
1523 Franklin Street
San Francisco, California 94109
Phone: 415-928-1100
Web: *http://www.iashs.edu*

Help for people with sex addiction.
Sex Addicts Anonymous
P.O. Box 70949
Houston, Texas 77270
Phone: 800-477-8191
Web: *http://www.saa-recovery.org*

SEX SUPPLIES: BOOKS, VIDEOS, TOYS

Adam & Eve, a retailer of adult products for more than 30 years: toys, videos, exotic lingerie, DVDs, lubes, lotions. On-line ordering, discreet delivery.
PHE, Inc.
P.O. Box 800
Carrboro, North Carolina 27510
Phone: 1-800-293-4654
Phone: 919.644.1212
Web: *http://www.adameve.com*

Products, supplies, workshops and instruction in tantra.
Tantric Temple

Phone: 718-899-2267
E-mail: *Carla@TantraNewYork.com*
Web: *http://www.tantranewyork.com*

Penis amulets and other magical amulets, talismans,
information, and supplies.
Lucky Mojo Curio Company
6632 Covey Road
Forestville, California 95436
Phone: 707-887-1521
Fax: 707-887-7128
Web: *http://www.luckymojo.com/penisamulets.html*

TAOIST SEXUAL TECHNIQUES
Mantak Chia
Author and Teacher of Taoist Sexual Techniques
Universal Tao Center
Tao Garden Health Resort
274 Moo 7 Laung Nua, Doi Saket, Chiang Mai 50220
Thailand
Phone: (+66)(53) 495-596, 865-035 Fax 495-852
Fax From North America: (1) (212) 504-8116
Fax From Europe: (+31) (20) 1524-1374
E-mail: *info@tao-garden.com or universaltao@universal-*
tao.com
Web: *http://www.tao-garden.com* and *www.universal-*
tao.com

VENUES PROVIDED BY THE AUTHOR
Ecotravel adventures to pristine, indigenous areas of Jamaica,
Costa Rica, and Belize.
EcoTours For Cures, The Education Vacation
Tour Leaders:
Eugene R. Zampieron, N.D., AHG, Ethnobotanist
Ellen Kamhi, Ph.D., R.N.— The Natural Nurse
Jamba Maroon, Bush Doctor
Kibret Neguse, Musician
P.O. Box 525
Oyster Bay, New York 11771
Phone: 800-829-0918
Web: *http://www.naturalnurse.com*

Ongoing one-day seminars in New York City's
Chinatown, with a focus on Chinese herbology.
Understanding Chinese Medicine: A Personalized Tour of
Chinatown, New York City
P.O. Box 525
Oyster Bay, New York 11771
Phone: 800-829-0918

WATER FILTRATION, AIR PURIFICATION, AND ENVIRONMENTAL SCREENING TESTS FOR TOXIC EXPOSURE, ALLERGIES
Environmental Detoxification Consultants & Products
P.O. Box 525
Oyster Bay, New York 11771
Phone: 800-829-0918
E-mail: *ezkpz@juno.com*

Contributors

Eugene R. Zampieron, N.D., AHG

Dr. Eugene R. Zampieron, N.D., AHG, is a licensed naturopathic physician, obtaining his Doctoral Degree in Naturopathic Medicine from Bastyr University in Seattle, WA., and is a Professor at the University of Bridgeport, College of Naturopathic Medicine. He is also a syndicated radio and multimedia host and Co-Executive of Natural Alternatives Health, Educational, and Multimedia Services, Inc. Along with business partner Ellen Kamhi, Dr. Zampieron is co-author of *The Natural Medicine Chest*, and *Arthritis, The Alternative Medicine Definitive Guide*. The duo also produce several syndicated radio programs, appear on T.V. regularly, and run Eco-Tours for Cures, which hosts excursions to Jamaica, Costa Rica, Belize, and New York's China Town to experience indigenous cultures, with an emphasis on natural healing.

Eugene Zampieron, N.D., AHG
203-263-2970
Web: *http://www.drznaturally.com*

Steven Angel, B.A., D.C.

Dr. Steven Angel, B.A., D.C., has been actively involved in researching the healing power of sound and music for more than 25 years. Dr. Angel presented his research to the First International Conference on Holistic Health and Medicine in Bangalore, India in 1989. Dr. Angel's research is discussed in the book *Mystic Souls*, by Lynn Halper.

Angel Holistic Healing Center
Phone: 516-897-5535
E-mail: *drangel777@yahoo.com*
Web: *http://www.chirosonics.org*

Lois Posner, R.N., LMT

Lois Posner, R.N., LMT, is a nurse educator with more than 25 years experience in teaching and practice in self-healing and energy cultivation techniques. She is certified by Mantak Chia in the Healing Tao System. Lois Posner serves as the managing director of Massage on The Run Wholistic Center.

Massage On The Run Wholistic Center
22 Wall Street
Huntington, New York 11743
Phone: 631-351-9898
Web: *http://www.massageontherun.net*

ABOUT THE AUTHOR

Ellen Kamhi, R.N., PH.D., H.N.C., The Natural Nurse®, is the coauthor of *The Natural Medicine Chest* (M. Evans), *Arthritis, The Alternative Medicine Definitive Guide* (alternativemedicine.com books), and author of *Cycles of Life, Herbs for Women* (M. Evans). She is a professional member of the American Herbalists Guild (AHG), is Nationally Board Certified as a Holistic Nurse (HNC), is on the advisory board of The American Association of Integrative Medicine, and is an appointed clinical instructor in the Department of Family Medicine at Stony Brook University.

Dr. Kamhi has been involved in the field of Natural Medicine for more than 30 years. She attended Rutgers and Cornell University, and sat on the Panel of Traditional Medicine at Columbia Presbyterian Medical School. She regularly appears on national T.V. and radio, and can be heard on WUSB (*www.wusb.org*) every Friday 6–7 P.M. EST. Ellen Kamhi has a private practice in Long Island and is a frequent speaker at conventions.

Index

Acknowledgments

Author acknowledgments

Blessings always to my parents, Sondra and Julius Kamhi; if they did not enjoy sex together I would not be writing this book! To my wonderful children, Brenda Soona Marie, Titus, and Ali; they are my most profound contribution to life on this planet. To my business partner and cofounder of Natural Alternatives, Health Education, and Multimedia Services, Eugene Zampieron, N.D., for his ongoing friendship and professional collaboration, I give my eternal thanks and blessings to our association. Love always to Michael Berman, my life partner, who literally sat next to me during the typing of this entire manuscript, and also participated in the research and testing of all the sexual rituals and exercises discussed in this book—it has been fun! To the reader—blessings on your path to health, happiness, and energetic knowledge; may truth and wisdom abound! And to God almighty, for blessing me with a wonderful life!

Picture credits

CORBIS:
p.101 Mark Hanauer; p.115 Larry Williams

GETTY-IMAGES/STONE:
p.51 Bruce Ayres; p.75 Elke Selzle

Additional photography:
Peter Pugh-Cook

The author would like to thank the Kabbalah Center, New York, for their kind permission to reproduce the sacred symbol on page 66.